Kinesiology Laboratory Manual for Physical Therapist Assistants

Kinesiology Laboratory Manual for Physical Therapist Assistants

Mary Alice Duesterhaus Minor, MS, PT

Program Director
Physical Therapist Assistant Program
Sanford-Brown College
St. Louis, Missouri

Lynn S. Lippert, MS, PT

Program Director
Physical Therapist Assistant Program
Mt. Hood Community College
Gresham, Oregon

with contributions by

Scott Duesterhaus Minor, PhD, PT

Program in Physical Therapy
Washington University School of Medicine
St. Louis, Missouri

 F. A. Davis Company • Philadelphia

F. A. Davis Company
1915 Arch Street
Philadelphia, PA 19103

Printed in Canada

Last digit indicates print number: 10 9 8 7 6 5 4 3 2 2

Publisher: Jean-François Vilain
Developmental Editor: Crystal Spraggins
Production Editor: Stephen D. Johnson
Cover Designer: Louis J. Forgione

As new scientific information becomes available through basic and clinical research, recommended treatments and drug therapies undergo changes. The authors and publisher have done everything possible to make this book accurate, up to date, and in accord with accepted standards at the time of publication. The authors, editors, and publisher are not responsible for errors or omissions or for consequences from application of the book, and make no warranty, expressed or implied, in regard to the contents of the book. Any practice described in this book should be applied by the reader in accordance with professional standards of care used in regard to the unique circumstances that may apply in each situation. The reader is advised always to check product information (package inserts) for changes and new information regarding dose and contraindications before administering any drug. Caution is especially urged when using new or infrequently ordered drugs.

ISBN: 0-8036-0203-0

DEDICATION

To the students who desire to learn so as to help others.

MADM

To Kate and Kellen, who promise to remain recognizable members
of the human race during their teen years.

LSL

PREFACE

This laboratory manual is designed to complement Lippert's *Clinical Kinesiology for Physical Therapist Assistants*, but it can be used with other textbooks as well. Each chapter of the manual is divided into three parts: Worksheets, Lab Activities, and Post-Lab Questions.

- The Worksheets are designed to assist the student in preparing for the lab session and should be completed by the student prior to class.
- The Lab Activities are designed to be completed in small groups as part of the lab session. The resources needed for the activities are those readily available and are not costly.
- The Post-Lab Questions are to be completed outside the lab sessions as a review.

We attempted to include the same key concepts in each chapter, as applicable, to allow the students to apply those concepts to a new body region.

The focus of the manual is on understanding normal kinesiology, and thus a selection of normal activities has been presented. We believe that students need to understand normal function before they can appreciate the abnormal. For this reason, the chapters on gait and posture, for example, include a general overview of the normal.

Arthrokinetic concepts involving the convex-concave law are included to provide an introduction to basic joint movements. However, by including this material, we do not mean to imply, suggest, or promote the idea that joint mobilization is an entry-level skill for physical therapist assistants. The concept of open-chain versus closed-chain activities, having gained popularity in the last few years, has also been included.

This manual is the result of many years of teaching kinesiology to PTA, OTA, and PT students. The authors test-piloted this version during development with the classes they were teaching. Student participation in lab sessions improved, feedback was positive, and suggestions were incorporated into the final version. We thank our students for their patience and their helpful suggestions.

MADM

LSL

ACKNOWLEDGMENTS

The first course I taught in my first teaching job was kinesiology. I was not comfortable because I knew that I did not have the grasp of the content needed to teach this important foundation course. I grew. I met my husband as a result of wanting someone else to teach kinesiology. The second time I taught kinesiology was as a team with Scott. Over the years, kinesiology has become one of my preferred courses to teach. Now, through the desire to write a lab manual for kinesiology, I have been given the opportunity to work with Lynn Lippert, which has been a pleasant learning experience. From Lynn I have learned to be even more organized and to be a better instructor of kinesiology. Thanks Lynn. Sarah, thanks for your patience when I needed to work on "the book" instead of doing something for you. Thanks to Maggie Clabough, PTA, for your input and support. Thanks to Jean-François Vilain, Publisher, Health Professions, for F. A. Davis, for bringing Lynn and me together and for supporting this project. Thanks to Crystal Spraggins, Developmental Editor, and Robert Butler, Assistant Director of Production, for translating our ideas into such a fine final format.

MADM

I agree with those who believe that it takes a village to raise a child. I also believe that it takes almost that many people to write a book. Sal Jepson offered editorial suggestions, fed the llamas during much of this project, and contributed many of her illustrations from the Lippert text. Joyce Shields, LPTA, contributed her artistic talent and positive energy to many of the illustrations. Our students "field tested" this manual and offered many useful suggestions. Mary Alice Minor is a woman of great patience and with whom I have learned. Both Scott and she have shown me new ways of looking at things.

LSL

Thanks also to those at F. A. Davis who have made this happen: Jean-François Vilain, Publisher, Health Professions, for believing in this project; Crystal Spraggins, Developmental Editor, is to be commended for her patience, her tactful way of saying, "Boy, is that a dumb idea," and her ability to follow up with a helpful suggestion. Stephen Johnson, Production Editor, and Robert Butler, Assistant Director of Production, have also been quite patient and have come to accept hearing "just one more little change." Ona Kosmos, Editorial Assistant, has been the one who always knew where everyone was and in what time zone. A special thanks to our "village."

MADM and LSL

REVIEWERS

Nancy Chandler, MPH, PT

Program Coordinator
Physical Therapist Assistant Program
Kennebec Valley Technical College
Fairfield, Maine

Joseph D. Cracraft, PhD, PT

Program Director
Physical Therapist Assistant Program
Community College of Southern Nevada
Las Vegas, Nevada

Lynda W. Jack, MS, PT

Academic Coordinator of Clinical Education
Department of Physical Therapy
Florida Gulf Coast University
Fort Myers, Florida

Julie Ann Muertz, MEd, PT

Instructor and ACCE
Physical Therapist Assistant Program
Belleville Area College
Belleville, Illinois

J. D. Wenderborn, PT, BS, MS

Coordinator
Physical Therapist Assistant Program
Laredo Community College
Laredo, Texas

CONTENTS

INTRODUCTION

Kinesiology is the science that deals with the relationships between anatomical structure and physiological processes that result in human movement. Knowledge of basic kinesiological concepts is fundamental to understanding the stresses placed on joints and joint structures when physical therapy exercises are performed. Movements of bones affect the motions of joint surfaces in distinct patterns. Interaction between bone movements and the associated joint surface movements can be therapeutic or damaging. It is important to apply fundamental kinesiological concepts correctly to achieve therapeutic results.

To examine human movement, several basic definitions used in kinesiology must be understood. These definitions demonstrate the interrelationship between structure and function. Definitions that are necessary for understanding and using the exercises in this laboratory manual and are not covered in Lippert's *Clinical Kinesiology for Physical Therapist Assistants* are presented on the following pages, with examples taken from the study of human movement.

OBSERVATION

Observation provides clues to movement. Methods of observation include both the tactile and visual senses. The tactile mode of observation is called *palpation*. Palpation uses the sense of touch to elicit information concerning bony landmarks; crepitus; muscle tone, shape, and size; skin texture and temperature; swelling; tenderness; and pulse. The visual mode of observation is called *visual observation*. Visual observation uses the sense of sight to elicit information concerning activities of daily living; skin color; gait; movement patterns; nail, scar, and skin condition.

The fingertips are used when performing palpation to find anatomical structures or determine skin texture. The fingertips are usually much more sensitive than other parts of the hand. It is important to know where to place your fingertips and how hard to press when performing palpation. Too little pressure does not convey enough information from the subject to your fingertips, for example, when a bony landmark cannot be found because insufficient pressure is used to sense the landmark through the overlying skin and muscle. Too much pressure obliterates the information to be conveyed to your fingertips and can be uncomfortable for the patient or practice subject. An example of applying too much pressure is when a pulse cannot be sensed because excessive pressure occludes the artery. The degree of pressure used during palpation can only be learned by guided practice and feedback. Occasionally the back of the hand is used for palpation, especially when palpating for temperature differences.

When performing visual observation, it is sometimes necessary to estimate joint position. Estimation of joint position requires establishing a reference point and estimating changes from that point. A method of establishing a reference point is presented in Figures 1.1(A) through 1.1(E). Figure 1.1(A) presents a stick figure of an elbow in full extension, when the elbow is straight. This position may also be called 0 degrees of elbow flexion. Figure 1.1(B) represents an elbow in 90 degrees of elbow flexion, such as when a subject has moved from the anatomical position with the palm forward to a position in which the palm is facing the ceiling. One-quarter of a full circle represents 90 degrees, placing the forearm at a right angle, or perpendicular, to the humerus. When the elbow is halfway between these two positions, 0 degrees and 90 degrees of elbow flexion, the joint position of 45 degrees of elbow flexion can be estimated, as in Figure 1.1(C). When the elbow is an additional 45 degrees beyond 90 degrees of elbow flexion, the subject would be in 135 degrees of elbow flexion. This can be determined, as demonstrated in Figure 1.1(D), by estimating an arc of 45 degrees

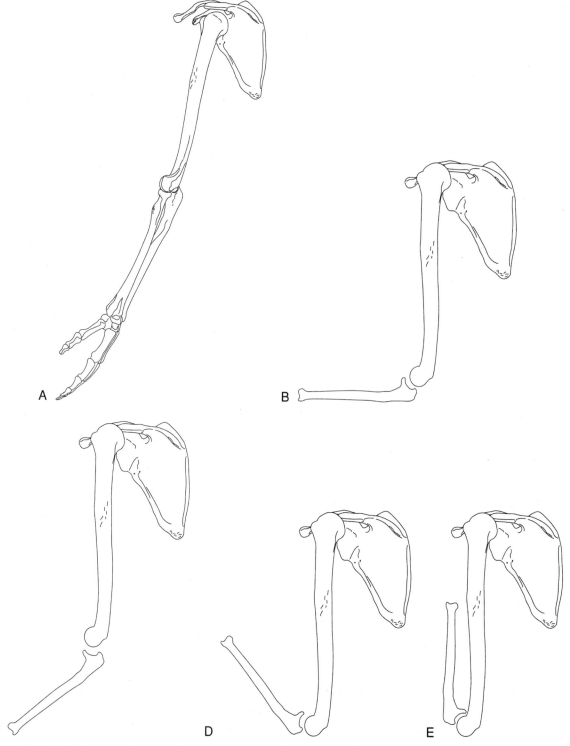

Figure 1.1 *(A) Full elbow extension, or 0-degree elbow flexion. (B) 90-degree elbow flexion. (C) 45-degree elbow flexion, the midpoint between 0-degree and 90-degree elbow flexion. (D) 135-degree elbow flexion. Calculated by adding an estimated 45-degree arc (as in C) to the quarter circle that represents 90 degrees (90° + 45° = 135°). (E) Hypothetical position of 180-degree elbow flexion.*

as in Figure 1.1(C), and adding it to the quarter-circle position that represents 90 degrees of elbow flexion as in Figure 1.1(B) (90° + 45° = 135°). For purposes of comparison, 180 degrees of elbow flexion, which should not be possible because of muscle bulk and joint structure, is presented in Figure 1.1(E).

STABILITY

The ability to maintain any given posture depends upon the interaction of the center of gravity, line of gravity, and base of support. The *center of gravity* (COG) is defined as the single point in the body upon which gravity acts. In other words, it is the single point about which all parts balance each other. This point varies as a person moves and changes posture or position. For a person standing in the anatomical position, the center of gravity is considered to be slightly anterior to the second sacral vertebra. When a person moves out of the anatomical position, the segments of the body are redistributed, changing the point in the body upon which gravity seems to act.

The *base of support* (BOS) is defined as the outer limits of support in a given posture. When a person stands in the anatomical position, the base of support is defined as a box shape outlined by the outer edges of the feet on either side, a line connecting the tips of the toes in front, and a line connecting the posterior part of the heels in back. A book lying on a desk has a base of support as large as the area of the book in contact with the desk. The book is stable and does not fall unless more than half the book is pushed over the edge of the desk. An opposite example occurs when attempting to balance a pencil on its point. The base of support for the pencil is extremely small, and the pencil has no stability and thus falls.

The *line of gravity* (LOG) is an imaginary line defined as the path that the center of gravity would take in falling if all support were removed, or if equilibrium were lost. The line of gravity may lie within the base of support or outside of the base of support. When the line of gravity is within the base of support, an object with rigid supports is considered to be in equilibrium (balance) and will be stable. When the line of gravity is within the base of support and there are no rigid supports, the object may collapse. An example is the legs of a human being. The joints of the legs must have muscle power present to keep the person from collapsing even if the center of gravity is within the base of support. When the line of gravity is outside the base of support, whether or not an object has rigid supports, the object will

attempt to fall. In this situation the object is considered unstable. When a human being is in a posture in which the line of gravity is outside of the base of support, the person can sometimes avoid falling by using muscle power. An inanimate object cannot avoid falling in this case because there is no internal mechanism, such as muscle power, to maintain equilibrium (balance).

BONY MOVEMENT

In kinesiology, a distinction is made between the movements of bones or limb segments (osteokinematics) and the movements of the joint surfaces at the end of bones (arthrokinematics). A *limb segment* is considered to be composed of the bones themselves. In the case of elbow flexion, the proximal limb segment would be the humerus and the distal limb segment would be the radius and ulna (forearm). Movement of a limb segment is described by the direction of movement of the bones in space. In the example of elbow flexion from the anatomical position, the forearm limb segment (radius and ulna) moves forward and upward, closer to the humeral limb segment. *There is a difference, however, between elbow flexion (osteokinematics) and the actual movement of the joint surfaces, that is, the concave or convex surfaces, of the elbow (arthrokinematics).*

Osteokinematics

The manner in which bones move in space as a limb segment is moved is defined by *osteokinematics*. Osteokinematics describes the movements of bones (or limb segments) in space, *without regard to the movement of joint surfaces* of the bones. Examples of osteokinematics include the limb segment movements of flexion and extension (hyperextension), abduction and adduction, and medial and lateral rotation.

Movements of flexion and extension almost always occur in the sagittal plane. An example of flexion is movement of the arm forward and upward at the shoulder from the anatomical position. This is called shoulder *flexion*. An example of shoulder *extension* is movement of the arm downward and back to the anatomical position. Regional differences in the use of some terms—for example, *extension* and *hyperextension*—are evident in this laboratory manual. In some regions of the country, continued movement of the arm backward (posteriorly) beyond the anatomical position is called *hyperextension*. In other regions this movement is considered a continuation of arm movement downward and backward, and thus is considered *extension*. Lippert's *Clinical Kinesiology for Physical Therapist Assistants* distinguishes between both terms. When terms used by your instructor differ from those used in Lippert's text and this laboratory manual, they must be clarified by the instructor.

Movements of abduction and adduction almost always occur in the frontal plane. An example of shoulder *abduction* is movement of the arm up and sideways from the anatomical position, away from the body at the shoulder. When this arm movement continues above 90 degrees to an overhead position, the arm movement continues to be called shoulder abduction, even though the arm is now moving back toward the midline of the body. An example of shoulder *adduction* is movement of the arm down and back to the side into anatomical position at the shoulder. When the arm continues past the side of the body, either anterior or posterior to the trunk, this motion continues to be called shoulder adduction.

The movements of medial (internal) and lateral (external) rotation and pronation/supination almost always occur in the transverse plane. An example of *medial rotation* is rotating the shoulder inward from the anatomical position so the posterior aspect of the elbow is now facing outward (away from the body). An example of *lateral rotation* is rotating the shoulder outward from the anatomical position so the posterior aspect of the elbow is now facing inward (toward the body). An example of *pronation* is rotation of the forearm inward from the anatomical position, while maintaining the upper arm in the anatomical position, so the palm is now facing inward (toward the body). An example of *supination* is rotation of the forearm outward as in the anatomical position, while maintaining the upper arm in the anatomical position, so the palm is facing forward.

The limb segment movements that do not fit this scheme for flexion/extension, abduction/adduction, and pronation/supination, and thus require us to say "almost always," are movements of the thumb and foot. These changes exist because of the differences in orientation of the thumb and foot in the anatomical position. Specifics of these variances can be found in Lippert's text, *Clinical Kinesiology for Physical Therapist Assistants*.

Arthrokinematics

When limb segments move in space, the ends of the bones—or joint surfaces—also move in space. Although a limb segment or a joint may be described as moving in flexion, extension, abduction, adduction, medial rotation, or lateral rotation, the manner of joint surface movement is *not* described in these terms. The manner in which adjoining joint surfaces move during limb segment movement is defined by *arthrokinematics*.

Because joint surfaces are curved and not uniform in shape, the manner in which different shapes of joint surfaces move during limb-segment movement varies. Almost all joints are a combination of adjoining joint surfaces in which one joint surface is *concave*, and the other joint surface is *convex*. A concave joint surface is rounded inward, much like a cave (Fig. 1.2[A]). A convex joint surface is rounded outward, much like a smooth bump (Fig. 1.2[B]). In some joints, one joint surface is a combination of concave and convex surfaces. The adjoining joint surface is also a combination of concave and convex surfaces. Such adjoining joint surfaces form *sellar (saddle) joints* (Fig. 1.2[C]). The combination of concave and convex surfaces from one joint surface match with the convex and concave surfaces respectively of the adjoining joint surfaces.

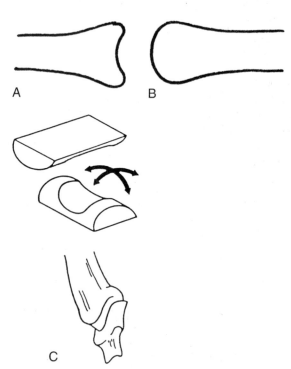

Figure 1.2 *(A) Concave joint surface. (B) Convex joint surface. (C) Sellar joint surface, combining components of both concave and convex surfaces. ([A] and [B] from Norkin, CC, and Levangie, PK: Joint Structure and Function: A Comprehensive Analysis, ed 2. FA Davis, Philadelphia, 1992, p 71, with permission. [C] from Swann, R [ed]: Body on file. Facts on File, New York, 1983, p 05.006, with permission.)*

Concave-Convex Law

The differences in shapes of adjoining joint surfaces require that the joint surfaces move in a specific way when their bones are moved in space. The specific definition of how concave and convex surfaces move as their bones move is stated in the *concave-convex law*. The concave-convex law describes two conditions that occur during limb segment movement.

First, the concave-convex law states that a concave joint surface will move on a fixed convex surface in the same direction as the moving body segment with which it is associated (Fig. 1.3[A]). An example of concave surface movement on a fixed convex surface is movement of the proximal phalanx (concave) joint surface on the fixed distal metacarpal (convex) joint surface. During finger flexion, the concave surface of the proximal phalanx moves in the same direction as the phalanx itself while moving on the convex metacarpal joint surface.

Second, the concave-convex law states that a convex joint surface will move on a fixed concave surface in the direction opposite to the moving body segment with which it is associated (Fig. 1.3[B]). An example of convex surface movement on a fixed concave surface is movement of the (convex) head of the humerus in a downward direction in the (concave) glenoid fossa. During humeral abduction, the convex surface of the head of the humerus moves in the opposite direction (inferiorly or downward) from the humeral limb segment (superiorly or upward) while moving on the concave glenoid fossa of the scapula.

To summarize the two principles of the concave-convex law:

(1) The *convex* joint surface moves in the *opposite* direction of the joint motion; and

(2) The *concave* joint surface moves in the *same* direction of the joint motion.

When performing passive range-of-motion exercises, careful consideration of the concave-convex law will help ensure that damaging joint surface motions do not occur.

Glide, Roll, and Spin

As adjoining joint surfaces move in response to limb-segment movement, the manner in which joint surfaces move can be characterized in one of three ways. *Glide* is the translatory movement of a joint surface in a direction parallel to the plane of the adjoining joint surface. An example of glide is the linear motion of a car tire as it skids on ice with the brakes locked (Fig. 1.4[A]). An example of glide in the body occurs when the femur moves anteriorly on the tibia without any change in joint range of motion. This action can occur when an athlete plants a foot to stop short, and the tibia stops while the femur continues to move forward.

Roll is the rotation of a joint surface about a moving mechanical axis. The joint surface undergoing roll moves across the adjoining joint surface. An example of roll is the normal motion of a car tire as the tire turns while moving the car forward under normal conditions of traction (Fig. 1.4[B]). An example of roll in the body is during knee extension as the femur extends on the tibia with the foot fixed. This action occurs when a basketball player jumps for a rebound from a crouch. As the knee extends, the femoral condyles roll forward on the tibial plateau. If posterior femoral glide did not accompany this type of roll, the femoral condyles would roll off the anterior edge of the tibial plateau during full knee extension.

Spin is the rotation of a joint surface about a fixed mechanical axis. The joint surface undergo-

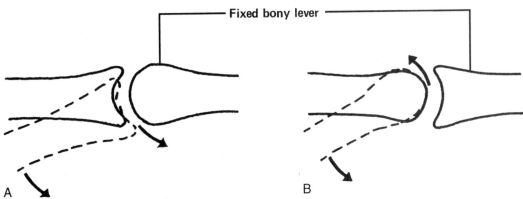

Figure 1.3 (A) *Movement of concave joint surface in the same direction as the moving body segment.* (B) *Movement of convex joint surface in the opposite direction from the moving body segment.*

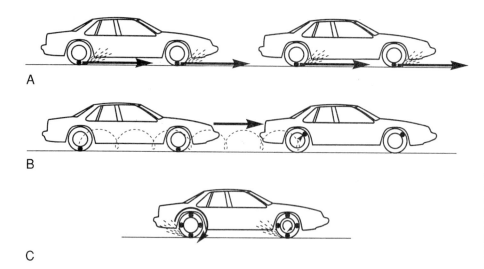

A

B

C

Figure 1.4 (A) Glide, represented by a car tire skidding on ice with the brakes locked. (B) Roll, represented by the normal motion of a turning car tire while the car moves forward. (C) Spin, represented by the spinning of a car tire on ice without gaining traction.

ing spin does not move across the adjoining joint surface. An example of spin is the rotatory motion of a car tire as the wheel turns on ice without gaining traction to move the car forward (Fig. 1.4[C]). An example of spin in the body occurs when the femur moves in medial or lateral rotation on a fixed tibia. This action occurs when an athlete plants a foot to make a sharp turn while running. When the foot is planted, the foot and tibia are fixed on the ground, and the femur attempts to rotate about its long axis on the fixed tibia.

For appropriate limb-segment motion to occur through full range of motion, glide, roll, and spin must occur. In the knee, the femur rolls on the tibia (or vice versa) during knee flexion and extension. There is enough flexion and extension in the knee, however, so that the femur would roll off the tibia (or vice versa) if glide of the tibia on the femur (or vice versa) did not occur in conjunction with roll. Therefore, in the knee, there must be a combination of glide and roll during flexion and extension movements. Because the condyles of the femur are different sizes, the medial and lateral aspects of the knee joint move at different speeds during flexion and extension. Therefore, there must be spin of the tibia on the femur (or vice versa) during the terminal 15 degrees of knee extension. Thus, the arthrokinematic qualities of glide, roll, and spin must all be available at the knee for appropriate knee range of motion.

Traction and Approximation

Joints at rest usually are not affected by large external forces, and the adjoining joint surfaces remain in a relatively relaxed position. The addition of external forces, however, can change the relationship of the adjoining joint surfaces.

When the surfaces of a joint are pulled apart, *traction* occurs, causing the adjoining joint surfaces to move slightly farther apart. An example of traction occurs at the shoulder, elbow, and wrist when a person carries a heavy briefcase in the hand while the arm swings by the side.

When the joint surfaces of a joint are pushed together, *approximation* occurs, causing the adjoining joint surfaces to press against each other. An example of approximation occurs at the hip, knee, and ankle when a person stands erect. The person's body weight from the thigh upward is pulled downward by the effect of gravity, and the lower leg is supported on the ground. Because the lower leg does not move, the weight above the knee presses the two adjoining joint surfaces of the knee together.

Traction can assist in promoting mobility in a joint. Approximation can assist in promoting stability in a joint. For patients with arthritis, traction and approximation must be used with care. A patient with rheumatoid arthritis will most likely find traction painful, although a patient with osteoarthritis will most likely find approximation painful.

END FEEL

The qualitative characterization of the feeling when a joint reaches the physiological limit of its passive range of motion is termed *end feel*. There are three major types of end feel. A *bony end feel* is characterized by a hard and abrupt limit to joint motion. This occurs when bone contacts bone (e.g., at normal terminal elbow extension) at the end of the range of motion. A *capsular end feel* is characterized by a hard, leatherlike limitation of motion with slight give. This occurs in full normal joint motion of the shoulder. *Empty end feel* is characterized by a lack of mechanical limitation of joint range of motion. This occurs when pain limits motion or upon complete disruption of soft-tissue constraints.

Besides end feel, there are two additional qualitative characterizations of the limitations of joint range of motion. *Springy block* is characterized by a rebound movement felt at the end of the range of motion. This occurs in the presence of internal derangement of a joint, such as torn cartilage. Soft-tissue approximation is characterized by asymptomatic limited range of motion. This occurs when the soft tissue of two body segments prevents further motion (e.g., at normal terminal elbow flexion).

The ability to palpate normal end feel and to distinguish changes from normal end feel is important in protecting joints during range-of-motion exercises.

MUSCLE MECHANICS

Effective Force of a Muscle

When a muscle works, it does so by developing tension in the muscle fibers. Although the tension is developed in the muscle fibers, the effective application of tension is to the bone segments at the points of attachment of the muscle (tendon). The tension is applied at both points of attachment, both proximally and distally. The total amount of tension developed in a muscle depends upon the size (physiological cross-sectional area) of the muscle fibers. The gross size of muscle fibers in a muscle and the gross number of muscle fibers in a muscle, which both contribute to size, are determinants of the amount of tension that a muscle can develop.

Whatever the size of a muscle, all of the tension generated in muscle fibers is not functional in producing rotatory limb-segment movement. When a muscle pulls in a perpendicular (right angle) direction with respect to the limb segment to which it attaches, the *line of pull* or *angle of insertion* is declared to be 90 degrees. In this case, all of the tension developed in a muscle produces rotatory motion. Once a limb segment begins to move, however, the 90-degree angle of insertion changes. When the angle of insertion moves away, either above or below 90 degrees, some of the tension developed by the muscle is no longer used for rotatory joint motion but causes joint traction or approximation. When the angle between adjoining limb segments is greater than

90 degrees, such as the example of full elbow extension presented previously (Fig. 1.1[A]), the tension developed by the muscle no longer produces only rotatory motion. Part of the resulting force at the joint will cause *joint approximation* because part of the muscle tension developed causes the adjoining joint surfaces of the elbow to be pulled together. When the angle between adjoining limb segments is less than 90 degrees, such as the example of 135 degrees of elbow flexion presented previously (Fig. 1.1[D]), the tension developed by the muscle no longer produces only rotatory motion. Part of the resulting force at the joint will cause *joint traction* because part of the muscle tension developed is causing the adjoining joint surfaces of the elbow to be pulled apart to a small degree.

Levers

The concepts and classes of levers are presented in Lippert's *Clinical Kinesiology for Physical Therapist Assistants*. The classes of levers are presented in Figures 1.5(A) through 1.5(C).

The biceps brachii muscle will be used as an example to demonstrate the relationship between classes of levers, center of gravity of a limb segment, effective force of a muscle, and direction of joint movement. The axis (A) of the lever system in this example is always the elbow. When the biceps brachii muscle works concentrically, the muscle acts as the force (F) that produces elbow flexion. The resistance (R) to elbow flexion is provided by the weight (created by gravity) of the limb segment at the center of mass of the forearm. The force (F) of the muscle is overcoming the resistance (R) of gravity. Therefore, the lever is defined in order by the axis (A), force (F), and resistance (R). This relationship, *A F R*, defines a *third-class lever*. In this case, the internal force of the muscle is moving the external load of the weight of the limb segment (which is created by gravity). The third-class lever system describing the biceps brachii muscle working concentrically is presented in Figure 1.6(A).

When the biceps brachii muscle works eccentrically, the weight of the limb segment (created by gravity) is the force (F) that produces elbow extension. The muscle acts as the resistance (R) that controls the rate of elbow extension. The resistance (R) of the muscle is working to slow down the force (F) of gravity acting on the center of mass of the forearm. Therefore, the lever is defined in order by the axis (A), resistance (R), and force (F). This relationship, *A R F*, defines a *second-class lever*. In this case the external force

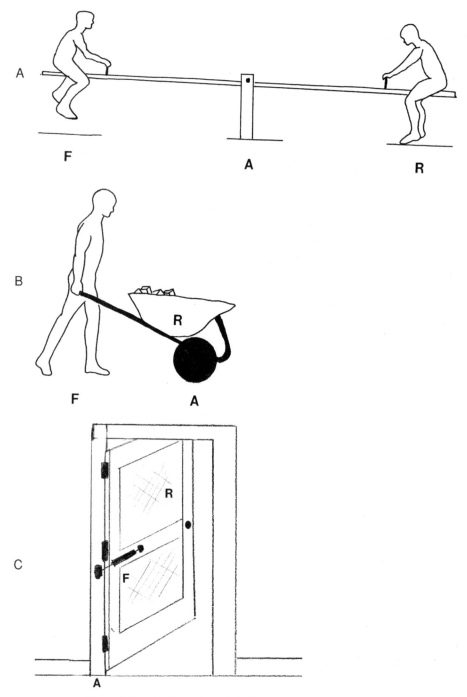

Figure 1.5 *(A) Class 1 lever. (B) Class 2 lever. (C) Class 3 lever.*

(F) of gravity is moving the limb segment against the internal resistance (R) provided by the biceps brachii muscle. The second-class lever system describing the biceps brachii muscle working eccentrically is presented in Figure 1.6(B).

Kinetic Chains

When limb-segment movement occurs as a result of a concentric contraction, muscles do not "know" if the proximal attachment (origin) is moving toward the distal attachment (insertion), or vice versa. When an eccentric contraction controls limb-segment movement, muscles do not "know" if the proximal attachment is moving away from the distal attachment, or vice versa. Muscles shorten during concentric contractions and lengthen during eccentric contractions without regard as to which attachment—proximal or distal—is fixed. There are, however, differences in

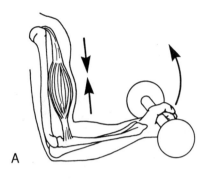

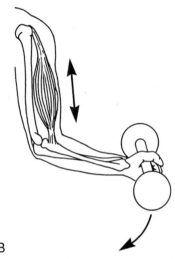

Figure 1.6 *(A) Class 3 lever. Diagram of biceps brachii muscle working concentrically. (B) Class 2 lever. Diagram of biceps brachii muscle working eccentrically.*

the effects of muscle contraction that occur when the proximal attachment is fixed than when the distal attachment is fixed.

The condition that occurs when the proximal aspect of a limb (entire extremity)—and thus the proximal muscle attachment—is fixed is called an *open kinetic chain*. An open kinetic chain is defined as movement that occurs when the distal aspect of a limb is free to move. This occurs when the *proximal* aspect of the limb is stabilized. Under this condition, the *distal* attachment of a muscle moves although the proximal attachment of a muscle is fixed. An example of this condition is contraction of the biceps brachii muscle to cause elbow flexion although the shoulder is held fixed and the hand is allowed to move. Under conditions of an open kinetic chain the distal end of a limb is free to move. Each joint of the limb is free to move in a relatively large number of ways. The effect of an open kinetic chain is a highly mobile distal aspect of the limb, moving on a stable proximal aspect of the limb.

The condition that occurs when the distal aspect of a limb—and thus the distal muscle attachment—is fixed is called a *closed kinetic chain*. A closed kinetic chain is defined as movement that occurs when the *distal* aspect of a limb is *fixed* and not free to move. Under this condition, the *proximal* attachment of a muscle *moves* although the distal attachment of a muscle is fixed. An example of a closed kinetic chain activity is performing a push-up in which the hand is fixed on the ground, and the elbow and shoulder move in a relatively constrained number of ways. This occurs when the distal aspect of the limb is stabilized by contact with the ground, or other constraining force. Under conditions of a closed kinetic chain, the distal aspect of a limb has relatively less freedom to move than does the proximal aspect of the limb. The effect of a closed kinetic chain is an immobile distal aspect of the limb, which limits, but does not totally inhibit, movement of successively proximal joints in the limb.

It is important to remember three basic concepts about kinetic chains. (1) An open kinetic chain occurs in activities in which there is relatively greater freedom of movement of the joints of the limb. The limb is usually engaged in an activity that requires mobility. (2) A closed kinetic chain occurs in activities in which there is relatively less freedom of movement of the joints of the limb. The limb is usually engaged in an activity that requires stability. (3) The definition of a closed kinetic chain requires the distal aspect of the limb to be *fixed* and not merely moving against a heavy load.

MUSCLE GRADES

There are a number of methods used to test the torque-generating capabilities of muscles (commonly called muscle strength). Manual muscle testing is a well-documented method used by physical therapists and physical therapist assistants. Two general methods of grading are used in manual muscle testing. Generally, grades given to muscles are based on:

1. The absence of muscle contraction (Zero or 0);
2. The ability to produce a muscle contraction that is detectable by palpation, but is not strong enough to cause joint movement (Trace or 1);
3. The ability to produce a muscle contraction that causes complete joint motion without resistance of gravity (Poor or 2);

4. The ability to produce a muscle contraction that causes complete joint motion against the resistance of gravity (Fair or 3);

5. The ability to produce a muscle contraction that causes complete joint motion against moderate manual resistance, but yields against maximal manual isometric resistance (Good or 4); and

6. The ability to produce a muscle contraction that causes complete joint motion against maximal manual resistance, or the ability to hold against maximal manual isometric resistance (Normal or 5).

From the two grading systems provided, it can be inferred that a grade of Fair (F)—or a grade of 3—is necessary for full movement against the resistance resulting from the effect of gravity. This is the least muscle capability that permits a person to move in three dimensions. Based on the definitions of muscle-testing grades, a person is placed in different positions when determining different muscle-test grades. Laboratory activities in this manual directing the student to palpate muscle origin, insertion, and belly, are designed to be carried out in the muscle-test position for a grade of Fair or 3. This means that these palpations are performed in a position that requires the muscle to contract against the resistance of gravity.

2

BASIC INFORMATION, SKELETAL SYSTEM, AND ARTICULAR SYSTEM

Student's Name _____ Date Due _____

WORKSHEETS

Complete the following questions prior to lab class.

1. Define:

Kinesiology _____

Biomechanics _____

Kinetics _____

Kinematics _____

Open kinetic chain _____

Closed kinetic chain _____

2. Match the following descriptions of bone markings with the correct term. Use each term only once.

_____ Projection above a condyle

_____ Rounded projection at the end of a joint

_____ Hole

_____ Spongelike space filled with air

_____ Tube-shaped opening

_____ Rounded projection beyond a narrow neck portion

_____ Small, rounded projection

_____ Large, rounded projection

_____ Sharp projection

_____ Very large projection

_____ Large depression

_____ Linear depression

_____ Ridge

A. Sinus
B. Tubercle
C. Crest
D. Spine
E. Foramen
F. Condyle
G. Groove
H. Fossa
I. Tuberosity
J. Head
K. Meatus
L. Trochanter
M. Epicondyle

3. On the drawing, label the parts of a long bone using the terms listed:

Epiphysis   Epiphysial plate   Diaphysis
Medullary canal   Endosteum   Metaphysis
Periosteum   Compact bone   Cancellous bone

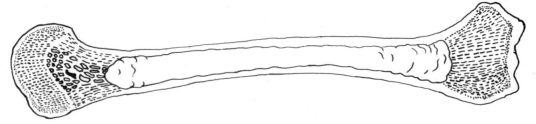

Figure 2.1   Long bone.

4. On the drawing, identify the linear motion and the angular motion.

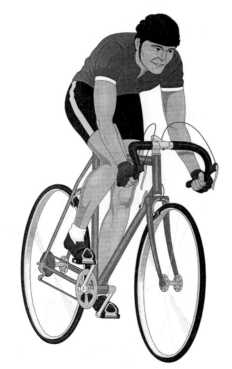

Figure 2.2   Bicycle rider.

5. Fill in the blanks with the appropriate information about the types of joints, amounts of motion allowed, structure, and examples.

Types of Joint	Amount of Motion	Structure	Example
Diarthrosis			
		Fibrous	Skull
	Slight		Vertebrae

6. Below each drawing, fill in the blanks regarding planes and axes.

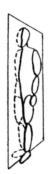

Figure 2.3

A. This is the _____ plane. It is associated with the _____
axis. Describe the direction of the axis: _____. List the motions that occur
in this plane around this axis: _____.

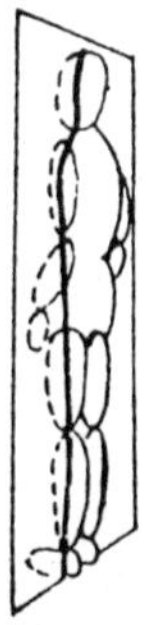

Figure 2.4

B. This is the _____ plane. It is associated with the _____
axis. Describe the direction of the axis:_____. List the motions that occur
in this plane around this axis: _____.

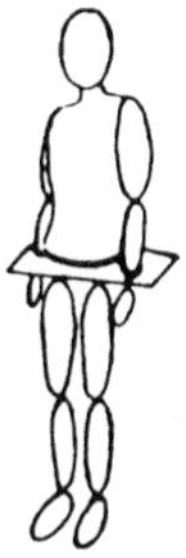

Figure 2.5

C. This is the _____ plane. It is associated with the _____
axis. Describe the direction of the axis:_____. List the motions that occur
in this plane around this axis: _____.

7. Match the following descriptions of a synovial joint with the correct term. Use each term only once.

_____ Enclosed cavity filled with fluid that prevents friction on moving parts

_____ Strong cord of connective tissue that attaches a muscle to another part

_____ The inside lining of the joint capsule

_____ Strong, fibrous connective tissue band that attaches bone to bone

_____ Flat, thin, fibrous sheet of connective tissue that attaches a muscle to another part

_____ Fibrous connective tissue that surrounds a joint

_____ Sheath of connective tissue that surrounds a muscle

_____ Fluid secreted from inside the lining of the joint capsule that lubricates the joint

_____ Smooth covering of bone ends

A. Joint capsule
B. Synovial membrane
C. Synovial fluid
D. Tendon
E. Articular cartilage
F. Bursa
G. Aponeurosis
H. Ligament
I. Fascia

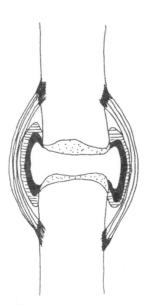

Figure 2.6   Synovial joint.

8. Label the drawing of the synovial joint using the following terms:

A. Ligament
B. Bone
C. Joint space
D. Synovial fluid
E. Synovial membrane
F. Articular cartilage
G. Joint capsule

9. Using the following descriptive terms, fill in the blanks to complete the sentences. Terms may be used more than once.

Medial	Superior	Proximal	Superficial	Anterior
Lateral	Inferior	Distal	Deep	Posterior

A. The tibia is the _____ bone of the lower leg, and the fibula is the _____ bone of the lower leg.

B. The ribs are _____ to the scapula.

C. The _____ end of the humerus is at the elbow joint.

D. The brachialis muscle lies underneath the biceps; therefore, it is _____ to the biceps.

E. The head is _____ to the chest.

F. The _____ end of the tibia is at the knee joint.

G. The great toe is on the _____ side of the foot.

H. Your eye is _____ and _____ to your mouth.

I. The radius is on the _____ side of the forearm, and the ulna is on the _____ side of the forearm.

J. The scapula is on the _____ side of the trunk.

K. The shoulder girdle is _____ to the pelvic girdle.

L. Skin is _____ to muscle.

10. Physical therapists and physical therapist assistants observe their patients from a distance using the senses of vision, smell, and hearing. When they use the sense of touch to observe patients, it is called *palpation*. During this course in kinesiology, you will use palpation and vision in particular to develop your knowledge of the normal human condition. Development of these senses is critical to providing quality patient care.

A. List some characteristics that can be observed while assessing a patient.

B. List which sensory modality is used to perceive the characteristic.

A. Characteristic	*B. Sense*
Example: Presence or absence of a wound	Vision
Skin temperature	Palpation

11. Match the following descriptions of motions to the correct term. The reference position is the anatomical position unless otherwise indicated. Use each answer only once.

_____ Pulling your scapulae together

_____ Moving your leg toward the midline

_____ Rolling your arm outward

_____ Moving your hand toward the thumb side

_____ Turning your foot inward

_____ A combination of motions causing your arm to move through a cone-shaped arc

_____ Moving your arm across the body at shoulder level

_____ Moving your hand down the side of your leg

_____ Shoulder motion during bowling back swing

_____ Turning your palm posteriorly

_____ Moving your arm out to the side

_____ The position of the knee in standing

_____ The position of the forearm

_____ Bending the hip

_____ Synonymous with wrist adduction

_____ Starting at shoulder level and moving your arm outward

_____ Moving your foot outward

_____ Moving your scapulae away from the midline

_____ Turning your arm inward

A. Flexion
B. Extension
C. Hyperextension
D. Abduction
E. Adduction
F. Supination
G. Pronation
H. Ulnar deviation
I. Radial deviation
J. Inversion
K. Eversion
L. Lateral rotation
M. Medial rotation
N. Lateral bending
O. Circumduction
P. Horizontal abduction
Q. Horizontal adduction
R. Protraction
S. Retraction

LAB ACTIVITIES

1. In a group, students perform the following active motions.

SHOULDER	Flexion	Extension
	Abduction	Adduction
	Horizontal abduction	Horizontal adduction
	Lateral rotation	Medial rotation
ELBOW	Flexion	Extension
HIP	Flexion	Extension
	Abduction	Adduction
	Lateral rotation	Medial rotation
KNEE	Flexion	Extension

2. Do the following activities, noting the speed and distance traveled by each person.

    A. Line students up shoulder to shoulder and instruct them to walk across the room keeping their line straight.

    B. Line students up shoulder to shoulder in the middle of the room and instruct them to walk in a circle with the student on the right end as the pivot or anchor.

    C. Repeat activity B with the student on the left end as the pivot or anchor.

    Compare the speed of movement of each student in activities A, B, and C. _____

    _____

    _____

    Compare distance traveled of each student in activities A, B, and C. _____

    _____

    _____

    What type of motion is activity A? _____

    What type of motion is activity B? _____

3. Perform the following activities:

    A. Stand up from sitting in a chair.

    B. Sitting on the side of a treatment table with a weighted cuff on the ankle, extend your knee.

    Activity A is an example of a (an) _____ kinetic chain activity.

    Activity B is an example of a (an) _____ kinetic chain activity.

4. A. Assume three positions or activities where the upper extremity (UE) is in an open kinetic chain and three positions or activities where the UE is in a closed kinetic chain.

   B. Assume three positions or activities where the lower extremity (LE) is in an open kinetic chain and three positions or activities where the LE is in a closed kinetic chain.

UE Positions

Open	*Closed*
Example: Standing	Hands on arms of chair

LE Positions

Open	*Closed*
Example: Supine	Standing

5. Using skeletons and models, find examples of the following bony landmarks. Describe where the landmark is found. Example: Trochanter: Proximal and lateral on femur.

LANDMARK   LOCATION

Foramen: _____

Fossa: _____

Groove: _____

Condyle: _____

Head: _____

Crest: _____

Epicondyle: _____

Spine: _____

Trochanter: _____

Tubercle: _____

Tuberosity: _____

6. Using the skeleton and models:

   A. Find examples of the following types of bones.

   B. Name an example of each type of bone.

   Short bones: _____

   Flat bones: _____

   Long bones: _____

   Irregular bones: _____

   Sesamoid bones: _____

7. Using the skeleton and models:

   A. Find examples of the following types of joints.

   B. Give another name used to describe the joint.

   C. List an example of each type of joint.

Type of Joint	Another Name	Example
FIBROUS JOINT		
CARTILAGINOUS JOINT		
DIARTHRODIAL JOINT		
UNIAXIAL JOINT		
BIAXIAL JOINT		
TRIAXIAL JOINT		
SADDLE JOINT		

8. Practice the following observation and palpation skills on at least two partners.

   A. Palpate the biceps brachii muscle belly and tendons—first, while the muscle is relaxed, and then, while your partner is contracting the muscle.

   1) Describe how you used your hands to palpate (e.g., fingertips, light pressure).

   _____

   _____

   _____

2) Describe what you felt (e.g., soft, firm).

_____

_____

_____

3) Did what you palpated feel any different when the biceps muscle was contracting?

_____

_____

_____

4) If so, describe the difference.

_____

_____

_____

5) Did contracting the muscle help you to find the tendon?

_____

_____

_____

B. Palpate the medial and lateral epicondyles of the humerus.

1) Describe how you used your hands to palpate.

_____

_____

_____

2) Describe what you felt.

_____

_____

_____

C. Palpate the patellar tendon—first, with the quadriceps muscle relaxed, and then, with your partner contracting the muscle.

1) Describe how you used your hands to palpate.

_____

_____

_____

2) Describe what you felt.

_____

_____

_____

3) Did what you palpated feel any different when the quadriceps muscle was contracting?

_____

_____

_____

4) If so, describe the difference.

_____

_____

_____

5) Did contracting the muscle help you to find the tendon?

_____

_____

_____

D. Palpate your partner's pulse at the radial artery.

1) Describe how you used your hands to palpate.

_____

_____

_____

2) Describe what you felt.

_____

_____

_____

E. Palpate the ulnar nerve on the posterior medial aspect of the elbow as it passes just lateral to the medial epicondyle.

1) Describe how you used your hands to palpate the nerve.

_____

_____

_____

2) Describe what you felt.

_____

_____

_____

3) Describe what your partner felt when you palpated the ulnar nerve.

_____

_____

_____

F. Posture examination is a visual observation. The patient's posture is compared to the normal or ideal posture. Symmetry and deviation from normal posture are noted. Because you have not studied posture yet, compare the second of the following two postures to the first, making note of major changes. Example: In the preferred standing position, your partner shifts a major portion of body weight to the left leg.

1) Observe your partner while he or she is standing erect with weight distributed equally on both feet, which are placed approximately 4 inches apart with the toes pointed forward.

2) Observe your partner standing in his or her preferred standing posture.

3) Describe any major differences between the two postures.

_____

_____

_____

POST-LAB QUESTIONS

After you have completed the Worksheets and Lab Activities, answer the following questions without using your book or notes. When finished, check your answers.

1. List senses used to observe a patient.

   _____

   _____

   _____

2. List the types of joints.

   _____

   _____

   _____

3. List three structures of the body on the anterior surface of the body.

   _____

   _____

   _____

4. List the components of a synovial joint.

   _____

   _____

   _____

5. Diarthrodial joints can be classified based on their characteristics. Fill in the blanks with the appropriate information.

Number of Axes	Shape of Joint	Joint Motion Allowed	Example
			Shoulder
		Rotation	
		Flexion/Extension	
	Condyloid		
	Saddle		
			Intercarpal

6. Check which motions generally occur in each plane about the axis of motion:

PLANES/AXES	Flexion/Extension/ Hyperextension	Abduction/Adduction	Medial rotation/ Lateral rotation
Sagittal plane Frontal axis			
Frontal plane Sagittal axis			
Transverse plane Vertical axis			

7. For each joint listed, indicate if active motion is available in each plane.

PLANE	Shoulder	Wrist	Hip	Knee
Sagittal				
Frontal				
Transverse				

3

MUSCULAR AND NERVOUS SYSTEMS

Student's Name _____   Date Due _____

WORKSHEETS

Complete the following questions prior to the lab class.

1. A *force couple* is defined as:

   _____

   _____

   _____

2. In the picture below, the person in the rowboat is controlling the boat using a force couple. In which direction will the boat move if the person exerts equal force on both oars in the direction indicated by the arrows?

   _____

   _____

   _____

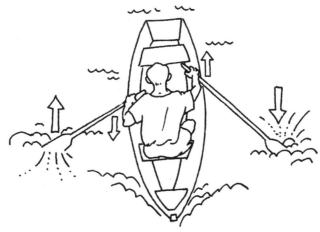

Figure 3.1   *Rowboat.*

3. When the muscles attached to the scapula (in the drawing below) contract, in which direction will the scapula move?

_____

_____

_____

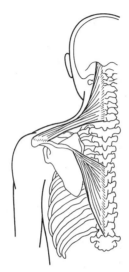

Figure 3.2 *Upper and lower trapezius muscles.*

4. Match the terms with their correct description of the movement of bones

_____ Joint movement on a plane parallel to the articulating surface

_____ Joint movement on an axis parallel to the articulating surface

_____ Joint movement about the axis perpendicular to the articulating surface

A. Glide
B. Spin
C. Roll

5. Fill in the blank with the term that identifies the movement of bones each drawing illustrates in Figure 3.3.

(A) _____ (B) _____ (C) _____

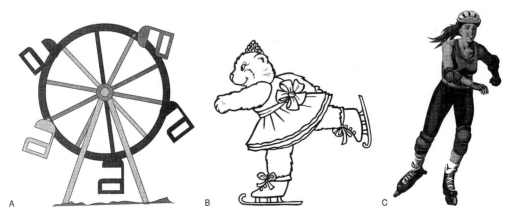

Figure 3.3 *Roll, spin, and glide. **(A)** Ferris wheel **(B)** Ice-skater. **(C)** Roller blade skater.*

6. Fill in the blanks using terms describing muscle attachments and function.

Attachment	Location	Open Kinetic Chain	Closed Kinetic Chain
		Stable	
Insertion			Stable

7. Using the terms listed below, identify the muscle shapes illustrated.

_____ Strap   _____ Fusiform   _____ Triangular   _____ Unipennate

_____ Rhomboidal   _____ Bipennate   _____ Multipennate

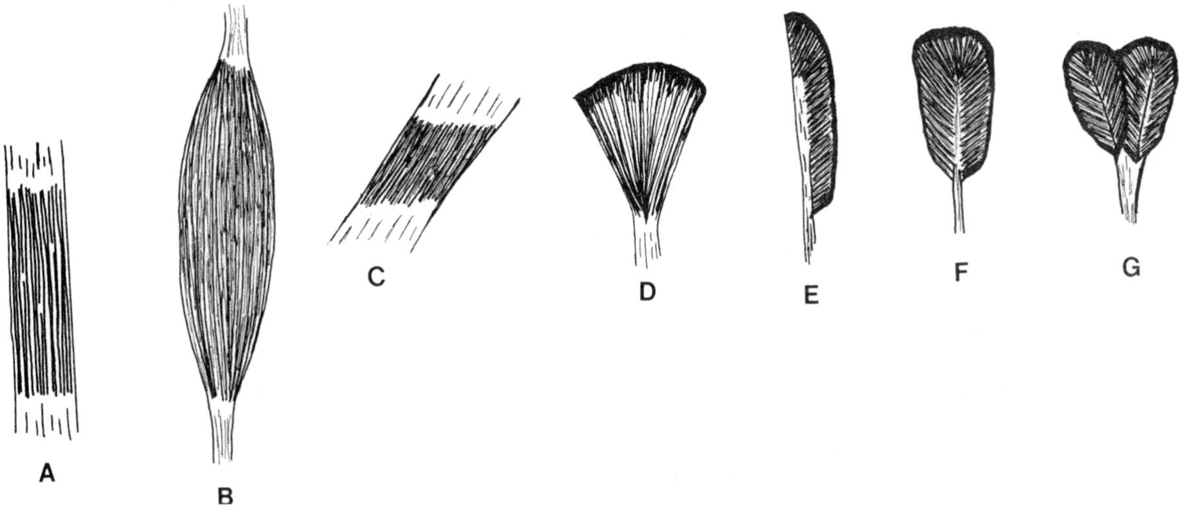

Figure 3.4   *Muscle fiber arrangements.*

8. Fill in the blanks with information about muscle fiber arrangement, direction of muscle fibers, and function.

Fiber Arrangement	Direction (Parallel/Oblique)	Greatest Potential (ROM/Strength)
Bipennate		Strength
	Parallel	
	Oblique	

9. Match the muscle characteristic with the correct description. Use each term once.

_____ Ability to be stretched beyond normal resting length

_____ Ability to receive and respond to a stimulus

_____ Ability to produce tension

_____ Ability to return to normal length

A. Irritability
B. Contractility
C. Extensibility
D. Elasticity

10. Match the muscle characteristic with the correct description. Use each term once.

    _____ Muscle is elongated over all its joints simultaneously, limiting joint motion at one or more joints

    _____ Muscle unable to contract in its most shortened position

    _____ Joint motion produced by passive insufficiency

    _____ Amount a muscle shortens from its most elongated position

    A. Active insufficiency
    B. Functional excursion
    C. Tenodesis
    D. Passive insufficiency

11. Match the type of muscle contraction with the correct description. Use each term once.

    _____ Resistance varies, velocity is constant

    _____ Resistance is constant, velocity varies

    _____ Resistance varies or is constant, velocity is zero

    A. Isometric
    B. Isotonic
    C. Isokinetic

12. Identify each type of muscle contraction as being either concentric (C) or eccentric (E).

    _____ Lengthening contraction

    _____ Shortening contraction

    _____ Insertion moves toward origin

    _____ Insertion moves away from origin

    _____ Type of isotonic contraction

    _____ Muscle contracts to move part against gravity

    _____ Muscle contracts to slow the pull of gravity on a part

13. Complete the statements using the following terms to fill in the blanks.

Agonists	Cocontraction	Nerve root
Antagonists	Dendrite	Neutralizer
Axon	Glide	Roll
Base of Support	Line of gravity	Spin
Center of gravity	Myelin sheath	Stabilizer

A. The part of the patient that is in contact with the supporting surface is the

_____.

B. The _____ connects the center of gravity to the base of support.

C. The _____ of the body is the point at which the planes of the body

intersect.

D. Sensory information is carried by the _____ to the neuron.

E. Information from the neuron is carried by the _____.

F. The _____ acts as insulation within the central nervous system.

G. _____ are the portions of the nerve adjunct to the spinal cord.

H. The shoulder girdle muscles act as _____ when one lifts a glass off the

table.

I. When a muscle acts to eliminate undesired motions during an activity, that muscle is

functioning as a _____.

J. Contracting the elbow flexors (biceps) and elbow extensors (triceps) at the same time is an

example of _____.

K. The muscles acting as prime movers of a joint motion are called the _____.

L. Muscles that perform the opposite motion of the agonists are called _____.

14. Check the motions that occur at each of the joints listed below.

Joint	Flexion	Extension	Hyperextension	Abduction	Adduction	Medial Rotation	Lateral Rotation
SHOULDER							
ELBOW							
WRIST							
HIP							
KNEE							
ANKLE							
GREAT TOE MTP							

15. Imagine playing on a seesaw with a buddy heavier than yourself.

    A. Where would your buddy sit in relation to the axis so the seesaw was balanced?

    _____
    _____

    B. Where would your buddy sit in relation to the axis so that you could easily hold him or her up in the air?

    _____
    _____

    C. Where would your buddy sit in relation to the axis so that he or she could easily hold you up in the air?

    _____
    _____

    D. Describe how each of these situations would change if your buddy weighs less than you.

    1) _____
       _____

    2) _____
       _____

    3) _____
       _____

16. On the drawing of the nervous system, identify and label the following structures:

Afferent neuron	Efferent neuron	Myelin sheath	Sensory receptor
Axon	Motor end plate	Node of Ranvier	Synapse
Dendrites	Motor neuron	Sensory neuron	

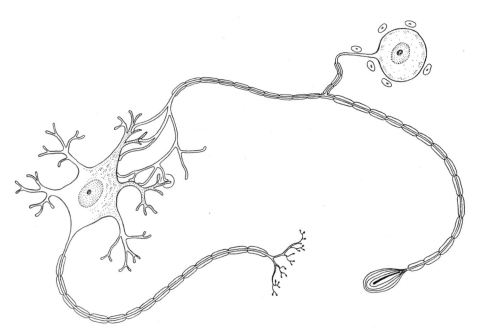

Figure 3.5   Reflex pathway. (From Magee, KR, and Saper, JR: Clinical and basic neurology for health professionals. Mosby-Year Book, Chicago, 1981, p 5, with permission.)

17. On the drawing of the brachial plexus, label the following structures:

Cords   Nerve roots   Peripheral nerves   Trunks

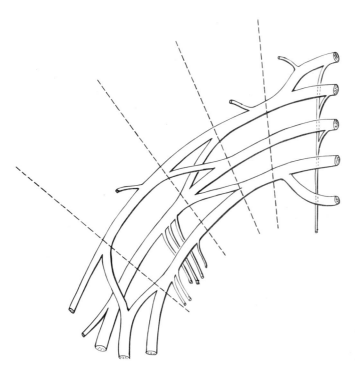

Figure 3.6   *Brachial plexus. (From Pratt, NE: Clinical Musculoskeletal Anatomy. JB Lippincott, Philadelphia, 1991, p 65, with permission.)*

18. On the drawing of the spinal cord, label the following structures:

Anterior horn	Motor pathway	Peripheral nerve	Sensory pathway
Gray matter	Nerve tract	Posterior horn	White matter

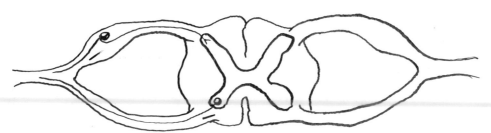

Figure 3.7   *Spinal cord.*

LAB ACTIVITIES

1. In a group, students perform as active motion the following motions:

SHOULDER	Flexion	Extension	Hyperextension
	Abduction	Adduction	
	Horizontal abduction	Horizontal adduction	
	Medial rotation	Lateral rotation	

| ELBOW | Flexion | Extension | |

| WRIST | Flexion | Neutral | Extension |
| | Ulnar deviation | Radial deviation | |

HIP	Flexion	Extension	Hyperextension
	Abduction	Adduction	
	Medial rotation	Lateral rotation	

| KNEE | Flexion | Extension | |

| ANKLE | Dorsiflexion | Plantar flexion | |

2. The following exercises are to be performed in the sitting position with the elbow straight.

   Perform shoulder flexion with a 5-pound weight held in the hand.

   Repeat with a 5-pound weighted cuff placed above the elbow.

   A. Which motion is easier to perform?

   _____

   B. Why?

   _____

   _____

3. Remove nails from a board, varying where you place your hand on the handle of the hammer.

   First, hold the handle close to the head of the hammer.

   Second, hold the handle close to the end of the handle.

   A. Which position is most effective?

   _____

   B. Why?

   _____

   _____

4. Standing with your back and legs against the wall, attempt to pick up an object on the floor 5 inches in front of your toes without flexing your knees.

   A. Could you pick up the object?

   _____

   B. Explain.

   _____

   _____

5. Stand with one foot on each side of a doorjamb such that your forefoot is beyond the door frame and your nose touches the door frame. Try to rise up on your toes.

   A. Could you rise up on your toes?

   _____

   B. Explain.

   _____

   _____

6. With your partner behind you as a spotter:

   First, sit in a wheelchair with your feet on the footplates and wheel up a ramp.

   Repeat with a backpack with books attached to the back of the wheelchair.

   Repeat, sitting tailor-style (Indian-style) in the wheelchair.

   A. What happened the first time up the ramp?

   _____

   B. What happened the second time up the ramp?

   _____

   C. What happened the third time up the ramp?

   _____

   D. Explain.

   _____

   _____

7. Repeat No. 6 using an amputee wheelchair. (If an amputee wheelchair is not available, add weighted cuffs to the footplates of a standard wheelchair.)

   A. What is different about the way the wheelchair handled going up the ramp in each circumstance?

   _____

   _____

   _____

   B. Explain.

   _____

   _____

8. Given that stability depends on the relationship of the center of gravity (COG) to the base of support (BOS), what happens when you reach for objects placed to each side and in front of you while in the following positions?

   Kneeling

   Heelsitting
   (From kneeling, lower yourself until buttocks rest on heels with knees still in contact with the ground.)

   A. Which position is more stable?

   _____

   B. Explain.

   _____

   _____

9. With your partner guarding you, keeping your feet together and without moving your feet, lean over and pick up an object from the floor placed in front of your feet starting at 1 foot from your feet and increasing the distance by 1 foot each try.

   A. At what point could you not keep your balance?

   at 1 foot ____; at 2 feet ____; at 3 feet ____; at 4 feet

   B. Explain.

   _____

   _____

10. To study the sensory distribution of nerves and the dermatomes, draw the distribution patterns on your arm and leg using a skin pencil. An alternate activity is to don a stockinette and draw on the stockinette the peripheral nerve distribution in red and the dermatomes in blue. The stockinette can be a permanent study guide. Refer to Figures 5–23 (page 69) and 5–25 through 5–35 (pages 72 through 80) in Lippert's *Clinical Kinesiology for Physical Therapist Assistants* for charts of sensory distribution.

11. Diagram the lever that describes *flexing your elbow* so you can touch your shoulder with your hand starting in the sitting position with the upper extremity in the anatomical position. Throughout this book many questions similar to this one are used. The solution to this one is presented to illustrate how to answer the remaining questions. In this sample the diagram appears more than once. In the rest of the book the diagram only appears once.

    A. On the figure, label the Xs that represent the axis, muscle, and gravity, and identify the specific joint and muscle group.

X	X	X	Direction of movement
Axis:	Muscle:	Gravity	
Elbow	Elbow flexors		
Joint			

B. Make arrows out of the vertical lines to indicate the direction of the movement, the direction of the pull of the muscle, and the direction of gravity.

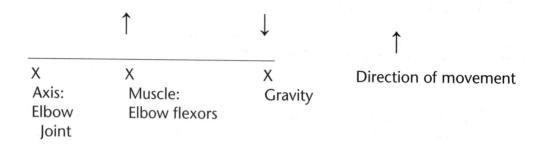

X   X   X   Direction of movement
Axis: Muscle: Gravity
Elbow   Elbow flexors
Joint

C. Identify the muscle and gravity as either *force* or *resistance*.
Generally, when the direction of the movement is the same as the direction of the muscle, the muscle is the force and gravity is the resistance.
Generally, when the direction of the movement is the same as the direction of gravity, gravity is the force and muscle is the resistance.

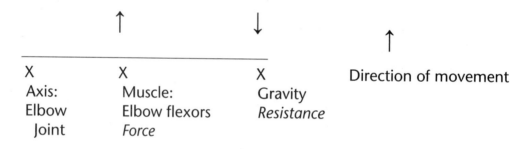

X   X   X   Direction of movement
Axis: Muscle: Gravity
Elbow   Elbow flexors   *Resistance*
Joint   *Force*

12. Analyze the activity of elbow flexion diagrammed in question 11 by answering the following questions.

A. Which joint motion is being analyzed? _____

B. Identify the "axis" of motion.

_____

C. Is gravity or a muscle the "force" producing the movement?

_____

D. Is gravity or a muscle the "resistance" to the movement?

_____

E. Which major muscle group is the agonist?

_____

F. Which major muscle group is the antagonist?

_____

G. Is the muscle acting to overcome gravity or to slow down gravity?

_____

H. Is the agonist performing a concentric or an eccentric contraction?

_____

I. Is the agonist performing an isometric or an isotonic contraction?

_____

J. Is the antagonist contracting?

_____

K. Is this an open or closed kinetic chain activity?

_____

13. Diagram the lever that describes *extending your elbow* from the position of touching your shoulder with your hand to the anatomical position of the upper extremity.

   A. On the figure, label the Xs that represent the axis, muscle, and gravity, and identify the specific joint and muscle group.

   B. Make arrows out of the vertical lines to indicate the direction of the movement, the direction of the pull of the muscle, and the direction of gravity.

   C. Identify the muscle and gravity as either *force* or *resistance*.

X   X   X

Direction of movement

14. Analyze the activity of elbow extension diagrammed in question 13 by answering the following questions.

   A. Which joint motion is being analyzed? _____

   B. Identify the "axis" of motion.

   _____

   C. Is gravity or a muscle the "force" producing the movement?

   _____

   D. Is gravity or a muscle the "resistance" to the movement?

   _____

   E. Which major muscle group is the agonist?

   _____

   F. Which major muscle group is the antagonist?

   _____

   G. Is the agonist acting to overcome gravity or to slow down gravity?

   _____

   H. Is the agonist performing a concentric or an eccentric contraction?

   _____

I. Is the agonist performing an isometric or an isotonic contraction?

_____

J. Is the antagonist contracting?

_____

K. Is this an open or closed kinetic chain activity?

_____

Refer to the information in the following table to answer questions 15 and 16.

Muscle	Location	Hip Action	Knee Action
Quadriceps	Anterior thigh	Rectus femoris: Flexion	All-parts: Extension
Hamstrings	Posterior thigh	Extension	Flexion

15. Lying supine with your lower extremity in the anatomical position:

Flex your left hip and knee through their full range of motion. Note the amount of range of motion available at each joint.

Have your partner passively flex your left hip while keeping the knee straight.

Flexing the hip with the knee extended is called a straight leg raise (SLR).

A. Did you have as much hip flexion motion with the knee extended as with the knee flexed?

_____

B. If you did not have as much hip flexion with the knee extended as with the knee flexed, where did you feel a stretching discomfort?

_____

C. In what muscle did you feel this?

_____

D. Explain what happened.

_____

_____

E. Is this an example of active or passive insufficiency?

_____

F. When an SLR is performed actively, what type of contraction is the knee extensor performing?

_____

16. Determine the maximum amount of left knee flexion that your partner has by passively flexing the knee with the hip flexed.

When your partner, lying prone with the hip fully extended, completes actively flexing the left knee as much as possible, answer the following questions:

A. Did your partner move through the maximum amount of left knee flexion that you noted when you passively flexed the knee with the hip flexed?

_____

B. If your partner did not move through full left knee flexion motion, attempt to passively flex your partner's knee by gently pushing the leg into knee flexion.

_____

C. Were you able to flex the knee more?

_____

D. If you were unable to flex the knee more, what prevented more motion?

_____

_____

E. Is this an example of active or passive insufficiency?

_____

F. If you were able to flex the knee more, what prevented your partner from actively flexing through the available motion?

_____

G. Is this an example of active or passive insufficiency?

_____

17. Starting with your elbow flexed to 90 degrees, forearm pronated, wrist extended, and fingers relaxed (slightly flexed), flex your wrist.

A. What happened to your fingers when you flexed your wrist?

_____

B. What is the term for this effect?

_____

C. Is this an example of active or passive insufficiency?

_____

POST-LAB QUESTIONS

After you have completed the Worksheets and Lab Activities, answer the following questions without using your book or notes. When finished, check your answers.

1. When the agonist is working to overcome the resistance of gravity, the part is moving in the opposite direction as the pull of gravity. Is the agonist performing a concentric or an eccentric contraction?

   _____

2. When the agonist is working to slow down the force of gravity, the part is moving in the same direction as the pull of gravity. Is the agonist performing a concentric or an eccentric contraction?

   _____

3. When an agonist is moving the part in the same direction as gravity but is overcoming an external force greater than gravity, is it performing a concentric or an eccentric contraction?

   _____

4. What type of contraction do the knee extensors perform when straightening the knee while sitting in a chair?

   _____

5. List general rules to increase the stability of an object.

   _____

   _____

   _____

6. Which drawing in Figure 3.8 illustrates the most stability in:

   The sagittal plane _____

   The frontal plane _____

   Both planes _____

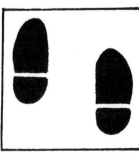 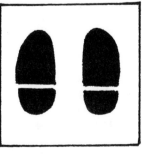 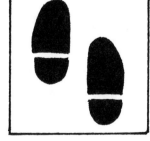

(A)   (B)   (C)

Figure 3.8   *Stability figure with feet.*

7. If you were standing facing the front when riding a bus, how would you place your feet to maintain your balance should the bus:

   A. Stop suddenly?

   B. Turn a corner?

8. In general, when standing how should you place your feet to provide the best base of support for maintaining your balance?

9. What happens to the COG when you pick up a 20-pound weight in your left hand?

   To compensate for the 20-pound weight, you shift your COG in which direction?

10. Where is the COG considered to be located in the body when you are in the anatomical position?

11. Identify the general location of the COG in the BOS in the following situations:

   A. You are sitting in a chair.

   B. You are a right unilateral below-knee amputee standing without a prosthesis.

   C. You are a bilateral above-knee amputee without prostheses sitting in a chair.

12. When an ice-skater coasts across the ice, the skate blades are an example of

13. When you open a door by turning the knob, the door knob movement is an example of

14. When a roller skater coasts across the floor, movement of the skate wheels is an example of

15. When the force arm is longer than the resistance arm, is it easier or harder to move the part?

16. Given the answer to question 15, which would be easier or harder to lift:

   A. A 5-pound weight strapped just below the knee?

   B. A 5-pound weight strapped just above the ankle?

17. For the implements illustrated, identify the class of lever. On the illustrations, identify the locations of the axes (A), the resistance (R)—the charcoal cube and the nut, and the force (F)—your grip.

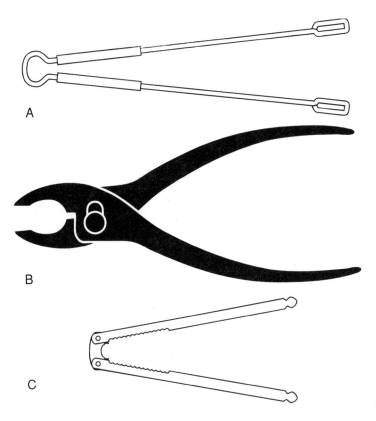

Figure 3.9 *(A) Barbecue tongs. (B) Pliers. (C) Nutcracker.*

Implement	Class
(A) Barbecue tongs	_____
(B) Pliers	_____
(C) Nutcracker	_____

4

SHOULDER GIRDLE

Student's Name _____ Date Due _____

WORKSHEETS

Complete the following questions prior to lab class.

1. On the drawings, label the following:

SCAPULA

Superior angle	Inferior angle
Vertebral border	Axillary border
Spine	Coracoid process
Acromion process	Glenoid fossa
Supraspinous fossa	Infraspinous fossa
Subscapular fossa	Infraglenoid tubercle
Labrum	Supraglenoid tubercle

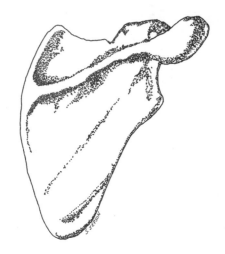

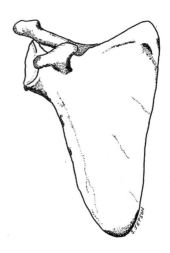

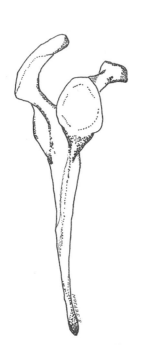

Figure 4.1   *Posterior, anterior, and lateral views of the scapula.*

CLAVICLE	Sternal end	Acromial end
	Body	
STERNUM	Manubrium	Body
	Xiphoid process	
RIBS	Ribs	

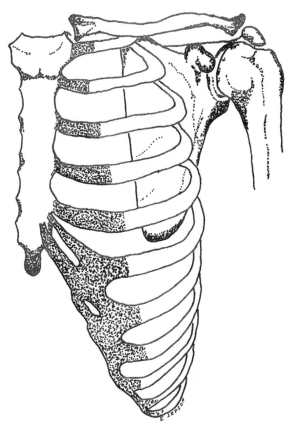

Figure 4.2   *Shoulder complex.*

SKULL   Occipital protuberance

VERTEBRAE   Spinous process   Transverse process

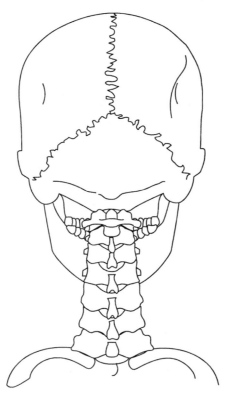

Figure 4.3   *Skull and cervical spine.*

2. On the drawings,

    A. Label the joints and bones.

    B. Draw the structures listed above the drawing.

BONES	Sternum	Clavicle	Ribs
	Coracoid process	Acromion	Scapula

JOINT	Sternoclavicular	Acromioclavicular

STRUCTURES	Sternoclavicular ligament	Costoclavicular ligament
	Interclavicular ligament	Articular disk
	Coracoacromial ligament	Acromioclavicular ligament

                Coracoclavicular ligament: conoid portion and trapezoid portion

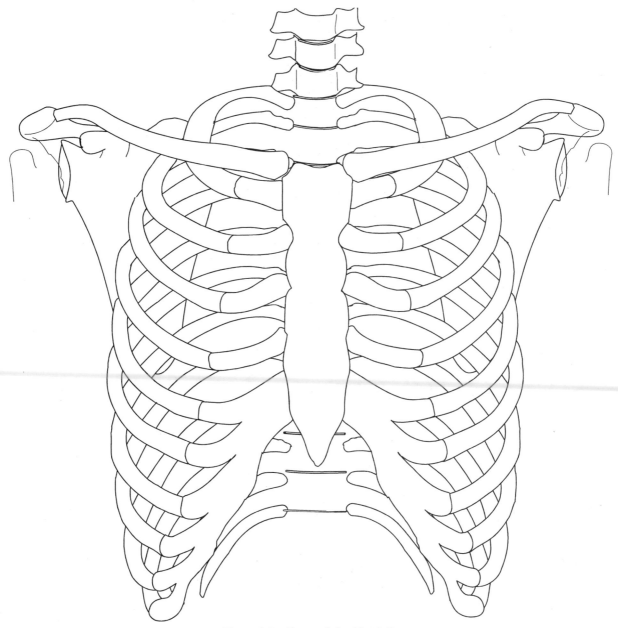

Figure 4.4   *Chest and shoulder girdle.*

3. On the drawings:

   A. Label the origin and insertion of the following muscles. Color the origin in red and the insertion in blue.

   B. Join the origin and insertion to show the muscle belly.

   Trapezius: Upper, Middle, Lower

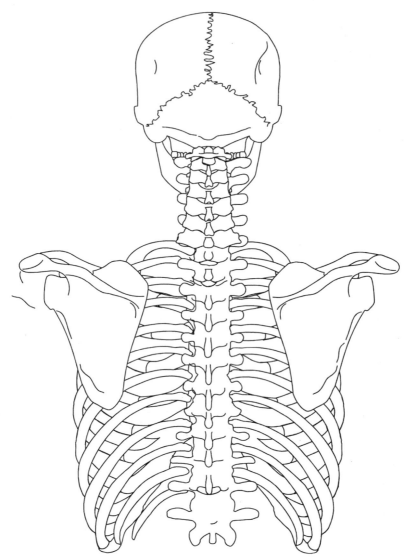

Figure 4.5 *Posterior view.*

Levator scapulae

Rhomboids

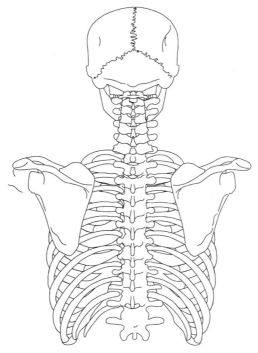

Figure 4.6 *Posterior view.*

Serratus anterior

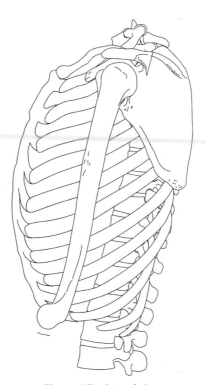

Figure 4.7 *Lateral view.*

Pectoralis minor

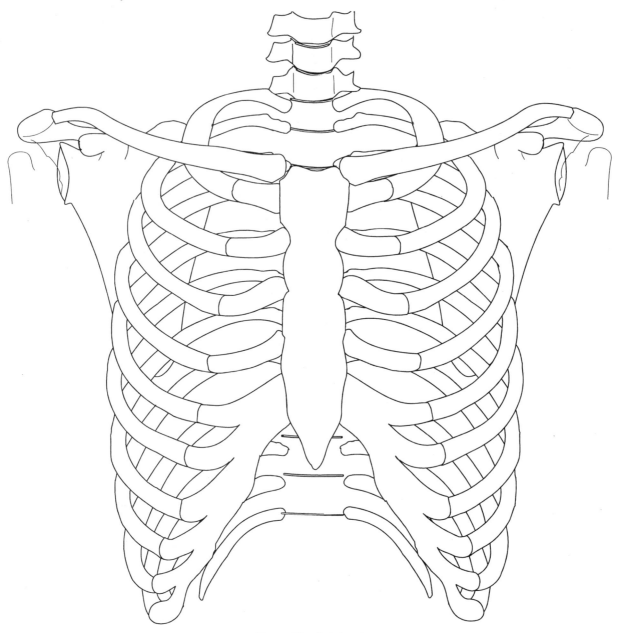

Figure 4.8 *Anterior view.*

4. Diagram the force couples acting on the scapula to produce scapular motions.

Upward rotation

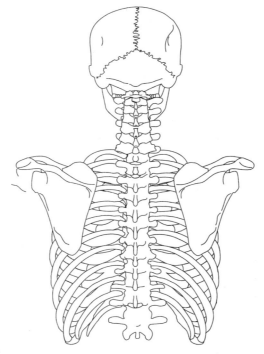

Figure 4.9

Downward rotation

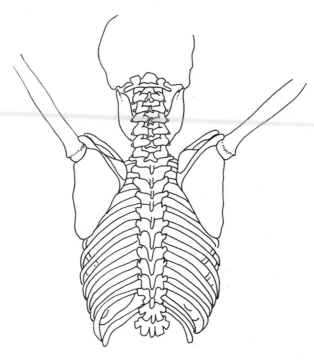

Figure 4.10

5. Identify the shoulder girdle motion demonstrated in each drawing.

   (A) _____   (B) _____   (C) _____   (D) _____

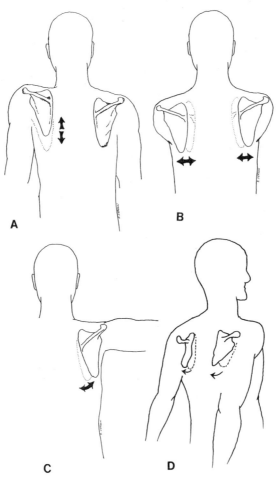

Figure 4.11   *Shoulder girdle motions.*

6. Match each ligament or structure to the appropriate function. There may be more than one correct answer, and answers may be used more than once.

   _____ Connects sternum to clavicle

   _____ Connects first rib to clavicle

   _____ Connects clavicles

   _____ Connects scapula to clavicle

   _____ Reinforces the capsule

   _____ Limits clavicular elevation

   _____ Acts as a shock absorber

   _____ Limits clavicular depression

   _____ Serves as roof over humeral head

   _____ Provides protective arch

   A. Sternoclavicular ligament
   B. Costoclavicular ligament
   C. Articular disk
   D. Interclavicular ligament
   E. Acromioclavicular ligament
   F. Coracoacromial ligament
   G. Coracoclavicular ligament

7. For each motion listed, check the muscles that are the major contributors to the motion.

Motion	Upper Trapezius	Middle Trapezius	Lower Trapezius	Levator Scapula	Rhomboids	Serratus Anterior	Pectoralis Minor
ELEVATION							
DEPRESSION							
RETRACTION							
PROTRACTION							
UPWARD ROTATION							
DOWNWARD ROTATION							

LAB ACTIVITIES
SHOULDER GIRDLE

1. On the skeleton, anatomical models, and at least one partner, locate, palpate, and observe the structures listed below. The reference position is the anatomical position. Having pictures for reference is helpful when trying to find structures. Not all structures are palpable on your partner.

Sternum: Located midline of the anterior chest wall.

    Manubrium: The superior portion of the sternum.

    Body: The middle and largest portion of the sternum.

    Xiphoid process: The inferior portion of the sternum. The most inferior part of the xiphoid process is called the tip of the xiphoid.

    Sternal notch: The indentation at the top of the manubrium formed by the right and left clavicle and the manubrium. Palpate the sternum starting at the sternal notch, and moving inferiorly palpating in turn the manubrium, body, and xiphoid process.

Clavicle: Located on the anterior surface of the trunk, superior and lateral to the sternum. Palpate starting at the sternal notch and moving horizontally, laterally and posteriorly along the clavicle to the acromioclavicular joint. Note that the medial two-thirds is convex and the lateral one-third is concave.

Scapula: Located superiorly on the posterior surface of the trunk between T2 and T7.

    Vertebral border: The medial edge of the scapula, which is approximately parallel to the vertebral column. Palpate from superior to inferior. Medially rotating the shoulder joint by placing the hand on the low back often causes the vertebral border to move away from the thorax.

    Inferior angle: The inferior point of the scapula where the vertebral and axillary borders meet.

    Axillary border: The lateral edge of the scapula. The axillary border, also called the *lateral border*, becomes difficult to palpate because the latissimus dorsi, teres major, and teres minor muscles cover the border. Palpate by moving superiorly along the lateral border of the scapula from the inferior angle.

    Acromion process: The flat broad expansion of the spine of the scapula that articulates with the clavicle and forms the top of the shoulder. The tip of the acromion is often used as a landmark for measurements of the upper extremity. The tip of the acromion is the anterior lateral aspect of the acromion.

    Spine of the scapula: A ridge or spine about one-third of the way down from the superior border of the scapula. The acromion process is the lateral end. The medial end on the vertebral border of the scapula is a flat smooth triangle called the *root* or *base of the spine* of the scapula. Palpate by moving posteriorly, medially, and inferiorly from the acromion process to the vertebral border.

    Superior angle: The angle formed as the vertebral border of the scapula joins the superior border. Palpate by moving superiorly from the root of the spine of the scapula. The superior angle is difficult to palpate because it is deep to the levator scapula and trapezius muscles.

    Coracoid process: The projection on the anterior surface of the scapula. Palpate from the anterior surface of the trunk inferior to the acromioclavicular joint. Deep to the pectoralis major muscle, the coracoid process can be palpated by pressing deeply into the tissues. This may be uncomfortable for the individual being palpated.

    Supraspinous fossa: The posterior superior aspect of the scapula above the spine of the scapula. Because the fossa contains the supraspinatus muscle, the fossa cannot be palpated.

Infraspinous fossa: The posterior inferior aspect of the scapula below the spine of the scapula. Because the fossa contains the infraspinatus muscle, the fossa cannot be palpated.

2. Locate the following muscles on the skeleton, anatomical models, and on at least one partner.

A. Locate the origin and insertion of the muscle on the skeleton.

B. Stretch a large rubber band taut by placing one end at the origin and the other end at the insertion of the muscle.

C. Perform the motion that the muscle does and observe how the rubber band becomes less taut, similar to the muscle shortening as it contracts.

D. Perform the opposite motion and observe how the rubber band becomes more taut and elongated, simulating the muscle being stretched.

E. After locating the muscle on the skeleton, locate the muscle on your partner. The position described for locating the muscle on your partner is the manual muscle test position for a fair or better grade of muscle strength. Not all origins, insertions, and muscle bellies can be palpated on your partner.

F. When possible, palpate the origin, insertion and muscle belly of each muscle by:

1) Placing your fingers on the origin and insertion and asking your partner to contract the muscle.

2) Moving your fingers from the origin to the insertion over the contracting muscle.

3) Asking your partner to relax the muscle, and again moving your fingers from the origin to the insertion over the muscle.

SITTING POSITION

Upper trapezius:	Located superficially on the posterior thorax
Position:	Sit facing away from the examiner with hands relaxed in the lap.
Origin:	Occiput and nuchal ligament.
Insertion:	Lateral end of clavicle and acromion process.
Action:	Shrug or elevate the shoulder girdle.
Palpate:	On the posterior aspect of the thorax above the scapula.
Levator scapulae:	Located on the posterior chest deep to the upper trapezius making it difficult to palpate.
Position:	Sit facing away from the examiner with the hands relaxed in the lap.
Origin:	Transverse processes of C1–C4 vertebrae.
Insertion:	Vertebral border between the superior angle and the root of the spine of the scapula.
Action:	Shrug or elevate the shoulders.
Pectoralis minor:	Located on the anterior chest wall deep to the pectoralis major.
Position:	Sit facing the examiner with the hand of the side being palpated resting on the low back.
Origin:	Anterior medial outer surfaces of ribs 3–5.
Insertion:	Coracoid process of the scapula.
Action:	Lift the hand off the low back. This muscle is deep to the pectoralis major.
Palpate:	Below the coracoid process.

Serratus anterior: Located on the anterior lateral chest wall deep to the latissimus dorsi laterally and deep to the scapula posteriorly.

Position: Sit with the shoulder flexed to 90 degrees.

Origin: Lateral aspects of first eight ribs.

Insertion: Anterior surface of the vertebral border of the scapula.

Action: Reach forward by flexing the shoulder while protracting the scapula.

Palpate: On the anterior lateral aspect of the chest wall.

PRONE POSITION

Lower trapezius: Located superficially on the posterior thorax.

Position: Lie prone with the shoulder abducted to approximately 145 degrees (in line with the fibers of the muscle).

Origin: Spinous processes of T7–T12 vertebrae.

Insertion: Base of the spine of the scapula.

Action: Lift the arm off the table.

Palpate: The muscle belly inferior and medial to the insertion.

Middle trapezius: Located superficially on the posterior thorax.

Position: Lie prone with shoulder abducted to 90 degrees and the elbow flexed to 90 degrees. The forearm should be hanging over the edge of the table.

Origin: Spinous processes of C7–T3 vertebrae.

Insertion: Acromion and spine of the scapula.

Action: Lift the upper arm off the table toward the ceiling.

Palpate: Lateral to the origin.

Rhomboids: Located on the posterior thorax deep to the trapezius.

Position: Lie prone with hand resting on the low back.

Origin: Spinous processes of C7–T5 vertebrae.

Insertion: Vertebral border of scapula between the spine and the inferior angle of the spine.

Action: Lift the hand off the low back toward the ceiling.

Palpate: Medial to the vertebral border of the scapula.

3. Scapular motion

A. Observe scapular motion as your partner flexes his or her shoulder. List the scapular motion(s) you observed.

_____

_____

B. Place one hand along the vertebral border. Palpate the movement of the scapula as your partner repeats shoulder flexion. Describe what you felt.

_____

_____

C. Stabilize the scapula to prevent its movement as your partner attempts shoulder flexion. Describe what you observed.

_____

_____

4. Observe and palpate as your partner performs shoulder abduction starting in the anatomical position.

   A. Describe the movements of the scapula and humerus in relation to one another.

   _____

   _____

   _____

   B. What is the name given to this combination of movements? _____

5. Work in groups of at least three members. Have one person stand erect. Have the second partner place a heavy weight in the first person's right hand, while the third member of the group palpates right shoulder girdle musculature.

   A. What happened to the shoulder girdle (e.g., elevation or depression) on the side holding the weight? _____

   _____

   _____

   _____

   B. Name any shoulder girdle musculature that contracted in response to the weight. _____

   _____

   C. Does the weight exert traction or approximation on the shoulder girdle? _____

   D. Is this an open or closed kinetic chain activity? _____

6. A. When your partner assumes the hands-and-knees position, what position does your partner's scapula assume?

   _____ Protracted   _____ Retracted   _____ Winged

   B. Is this an open or closed kinetic chain activity? _____

Student's Name _____   Date Due _____

POST-LAB QUESTIONS
SHOULDER GIRDLE

After you have completed the Worksheets and Lab Activities, answer the following questions without using your book or notes. When finished, check your answers.

1. List the muscle(s) of the shoulder girdle that attach to the ribs.

   _____

   _____

2. List the muscle(s) of the shoulder girdle that attach to the vertebral border of the scapula.

   _____

   _____

3. List the muscle(s) of the shoulder girdle that attach to the skull.

   _____

   _____

4. List the muscle(s) of the shoulder girdle that attach to the vertebral column.

   _____

   _____

5. List the muscle(s) of the shoulder girdle that attach to the clavicle.

   _____

   _____

6. List the joint(s) that make up the shoulder girdle.

   _____

   _____

7. Why is the scapulothoracic joint not a true joint? _____

   _____

   _____

8. What is the result of limited sternoclavicular motion on shoulder girdle motion? _____

   _____

   _____

9. Using the following descriptive terminology, fill in the blanks in the following sentences. Use each term once.

Medial	Anterior	Superior	Deep
Lateral	Posterior	Inferior	Superficial

    A. The spine is on the _____ surface of the scapula.

    B. The vertebral border is on the _____ side of the scapula.

    C. The glenoid fossa is on the _____ aspect of the scapula.

    D. The xiphoid process is _____ to the body of the sternum.

    E. The rhomboid muscles are located _____ to the trapezius.

    F. The coracoid process is on the _____ surface of the scapula.

    G. The upper trapezius muscle is located _____ to the levator scapula.

    H. The clavicle is _____ to the sternum.

10. Identify the following muscles:

    A. Attaches to the coracoid process: _____

    B. Attaches to the vertebral border of the scapula:

        1) On the posterior surface: _____

        2) On the anterior surface: _____

    C. Attaches to the superior angle of the scapula: _____

    D. Attaches to the spine of the scapula: _____

    E. Attaches where the spine meets the vertebral border: _____

    F. Attaches on the transverse processes of the vertebra: _____

    G. Attaches on the spinous processes of the vertebra: _____

    H. Attaches on the ribs: _____

11. Identify the following muscles according to their locations on the body:

    A. Which muscle is located between the rib cage and the scapula? _____

    B. Which muscle lies deep to the pectoralis major? _____

    C. Which muscle is the most superficial on the posterior upper back? _____

12. Name the muscle innervated by a cranial nerve: _____

    Name the cranial nerve: _____

5

SHOULDER JOINT

Student's Name _____ Date Due _____

WORKSHEETS

Complete the following questions prior to lab class.

1. On the following drawings, label the following:

   CLAVICLE

   SCAPULA
Glenoid fossa	Labrum
Acromion process	Coracoid process
Subscapular fossa	Infraglenoid tubercle
Supraglenoid tubercle	Infraspinous fossa
Supraspinous fossa	Vertebral border
Spine	Axillary border
Inferior angle	

   HUMERUS
Head	Anatomical neck
Surgical neck	Lesser tubercle
Deltoid tuberosity	Greater tubercle
Bicipital groove	Shaft

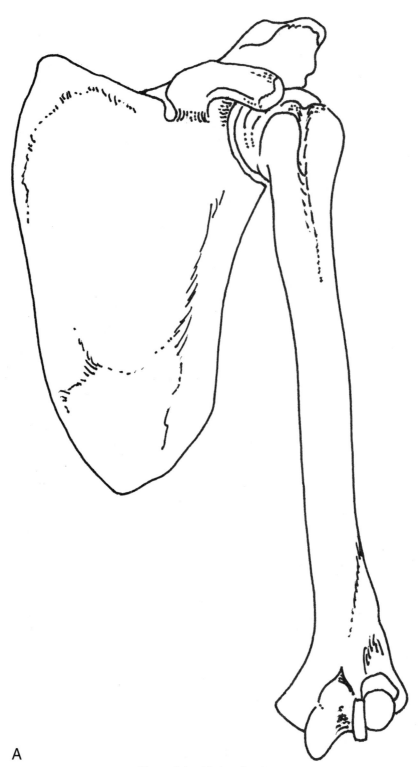

A

Figure 5.1 *(A) Anterior view.*

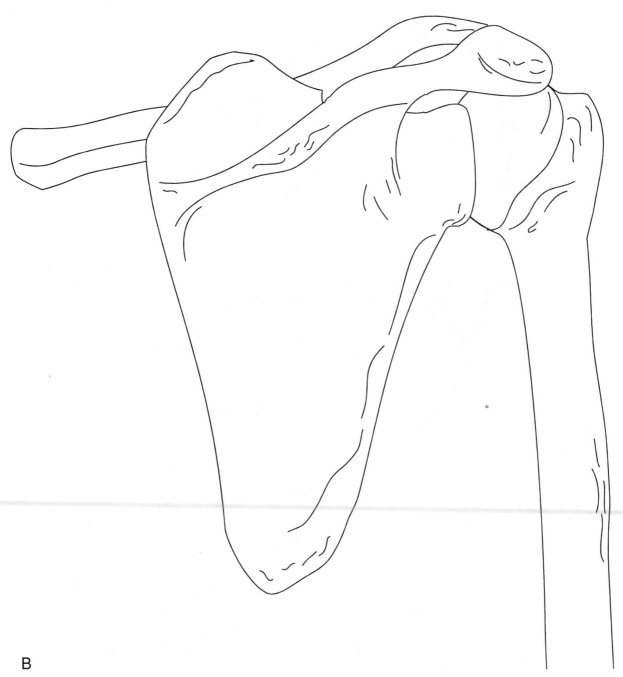

B

Figure 5.1 *(B) Posterior view.*

2. On the drawing,

    A. Label the shoulder joint and bones.

    B. Draw the coracohumeral ligament.

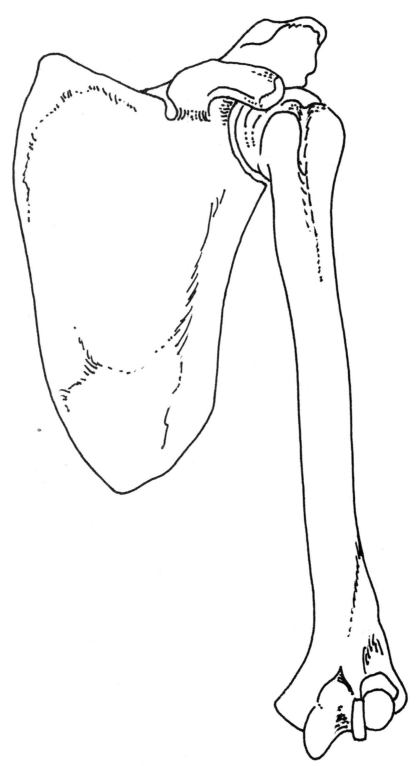

Figure 5.2

3. On the following drawings,

    A. Label the origin and insertion of the muscles listed.
       Color the origin in red and the insertion in blue.

    B. Join the origin and insertion to show the muscle belly.

Supraspinatus   Teres minor   Teres major   Infraspinatus
Proximal attachment of the long head of the triceps brachii

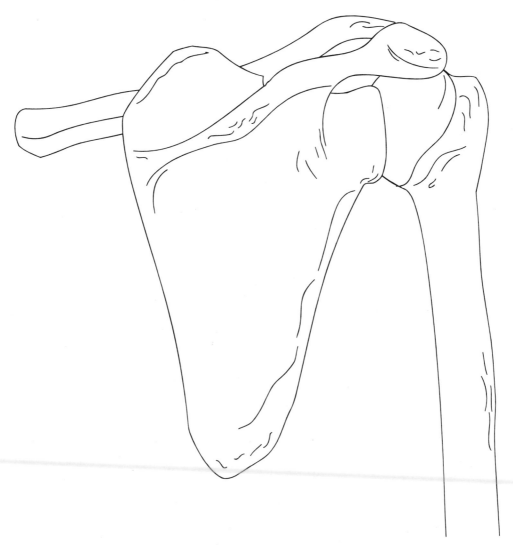

Figure 5.3 *Posterior view.*

Latissimus dorsi   Teres major   Posterior deltoid

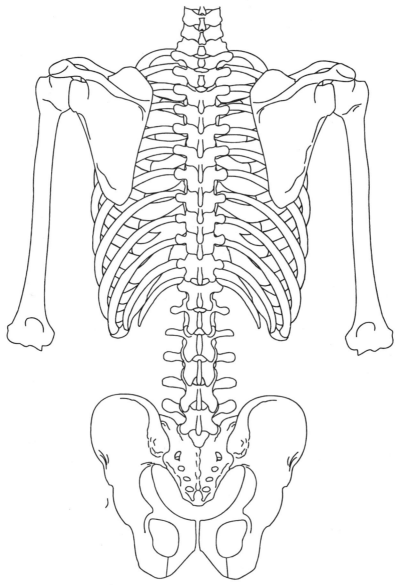

Figure 5.4   *Posterior view.*

Middle deltoid   Anterior deltoid   Posterior deltoid

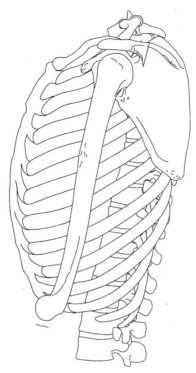

Figure 5.5   *Lateral view.*

Anterior deltoid   Pectoralis major

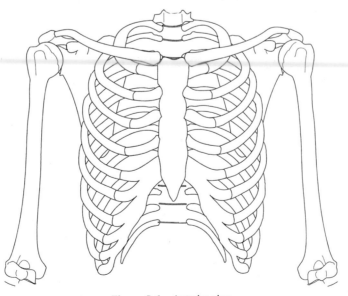

Figure 5.6   *Anterior view.*

Subscapularis

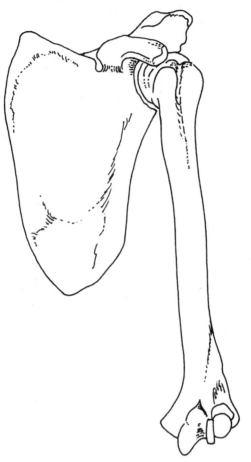

Figure 5.7 *Anterior view.*

Coracobrachialis   Proximal attachment of the biceps brachii

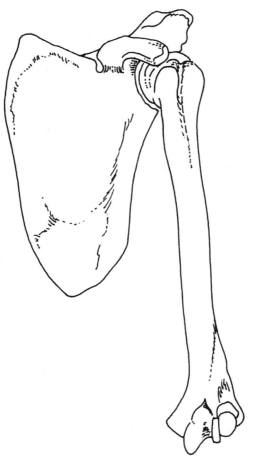

Figure 5.8   *Anterior view.*

4. Another name for the shoulder joint is _____.

5. Distinguish between the shoulder joint and the shoulder girdle by *listing the bones* of each.

Shoulder Joint	*Shoulder Girdle*

6. Distinguish between the shoulder joint and the shoulder girdle by *listing the motions* available at each.

Shoulder Joint	*Shoulder Girdle*

7. For the shoulder joint, identify:

Shape: _____

Number of planes: _____

8. For the motions available at the shoulder joint, indicate in which plane and around which axis the motion occurs.

Motions	*Plane*	*Axis*
FLEXION/EXTENSION/ HYPEREXTENSION		
ABDUCTION/ADDUCTION		
MEDIAL/LATERAL ROTATION		
HORIZONTAL ABDUCTION/ ADDUCTION		

9. Name the portion of the bone of the shoulder joint that is concave: _____.

   Name the portion of the bone of the shoulder joint that is convex: _____.

10. Match each ligament and structure to the appropriate function or characteristic. Use each answer once.

   _____ Provides attachment for the latissimus dorsi muscle

   _____ Deepens the joint

   _____ Keeps the humeral head rotating in contact with the glenoid fossa

   _____ Surrounds the joint

   _____ Strengthens the upper part of the joint capsule

   _____ Decreases friction between the deltoid muscle and the joint capsule

   _____ Decreases friction between the acromion process, the coracoacromial ligament, and the joint capsule

   A. Coracohumeral ligament
   B. Glenoid labrum
   C. Subdeltoid bursa
   D. Subacromial bursa
   E. Rotator cuff
   F. Thoracolumbar fascia
   G. Joint capsule

11. For each motion listed, check the muscle(s) that are major contributors to the motion.

Motion	Anterior Deltoid	Middle Deltoid	Posterior Deltoid	Supra-spinatus	Coraco-brachialis	Subscapularis
FLEXION						
EXTENSION						
HYPER-EXTENSION						
MEDIAL ROTATION						
LATERAL ROTATION						
ABDUCTION						
ADDUCTION						
HORIZONTAL ABDUCTION						
HORIZONTAL ADDUCTION						

Motion	Pectoralis Major Clavicular	Pectoralis Major Sternal	Latissimus Dorsi	Teres Major	Teres Minor	Infra-spinatus
FLEXION						
EXTENSION						
HYPER-EXTENSION						
MEDIAL ROTATION						
LATERAL ROTATION						
ABDUCTION						
ADDUCTION						
HORIZONTAL ABDUCTION						
HORIZONTAL ADDUCTION						

12. Describe the function of the rotator cuff muscles during shoulder flexion or abduction.

_____

_____

13. A. Which major nerve unit is located in the axilla? _____

    B. In relation to the head of the humerus that nerve unit is:

    ____ Anterior   ____ Posterior   ____ Superior   ____ Inferior

    C. What major blood vessel is close to this nerve unit? _____

14. Diagram the lever that describes *abduction of the shoulder joint* performed in the anatomical position.

    A. On the figure, label the Xs that represent the axis, muscle, and gravity, and identify the specific joint and muscle group.

    B. Make arrows out of the vertical lines to indicate the direction of the movement, the direction of the pull of the muscle, and the direction of gravity.

    C. Identify the muscle and gravity as either *force* or *resistance*.

X	X	X

Direction of movement

15. Analyze the activity of shoulder abduction diagrammed in question 14 by answering the following questions:

    A. Which joint motion is being analyzed? _____

    B. Identify the "axis" of the motion: _____

    C. Is the "force" producing the movement a muscle or gravity? _____

    D. Is the "resistance" to the movement a muscle or gravity? _____

    E. Which major muscle group is the agonist? _____

    F. Which major muscle group is the antagonist? _____

    G. Is the muscle group acting to overcome gravity or slow down gravity? _____

    H. Is the agonist performing a concentric or an eccentric contraction? _____

    I. Is this an open or closed kinetic chain activity? _____

LAB ACTIVITIES
SHOULDER JOINT

1. Using worksheet question 8 for reference, for each of the motions available at the shoulder joint,

    A. Place your open left hand in the correct orientation to represent the plane of a motion.

    B. Place your right index finger to indicate the axis of that plane of motion.

2. Knowing the amount of motion is important when assessing patient progress. There are standards for the normal motions for each joint. Being able to estimate the amount of joint motion available is useful. To begin to estimate the amount of joint motion, you must be able to identify these landmark degrees: 0, 45, 90, 135, and 180. The anatomical position is considered the 0-degree position and the starting position for measuring the amount of motion available in each plane. A right angle is 90 degrees. Halfway between 0 and 90 degrees is 45 degrees; 135 degrees is halfway between 90 and 180 degrees.

    A. Set the two arms of the goniometer at 0, 45, 90, 135, and 180 degrees.

    B. Without using a goniometer, place your partner's arm in 0, 45, 90, 135, and 180 degrees of shoulder flexion.

    C. For each of the motions available at the shoulder joint, estimate the degrees of motion available by checking the box that *most closely* describes that motion. (Do not use a goniometer.)

Motions	*0–45*	*46–90*	*91–135*	*136–180*
FLEXION				
HYPER-EXTENSION				
ABDUCTION				
HORIZONTAL ABDUCTION*				
HORIZONTAL ADDUCTION*				
MEDIAL ROTATION**				
LATERAL ROTATION**				

* Starting position: shoulder abducted to 90 degrees.
** Starting position: elbow flexed to 90 degrees.

3. On the skeleton, anatomical models, and at least one partner, locate, palpate, and observe the structures listed below. The reference position is the anatomical position. Having pictures for reference is helpful when trying to find structures. Not all structures are palpable on your partner.

   Scapula: Many of the landmarks on the scapula were described in the lab on the shoulder girdle. Refer to that lab if you are unsure of those landmarks.

   Supraglenoid tubercle: Located on the superior lip of the glenoid fossa. It is the attachment of the long head of the biceps brachii muscle. Located deep to the acromion process, the supraglenoid tubercle cannot be palpated.

   Infraglenoid tubercle: Located on the inferior lip of the glenoid fossa. It is the attachment of the long head of the triceps muscle. Located deep in the joint, the infraglenoid tubercle cannot be palpated.

   Humerus

   Head: The smooth semi-round portion of the proximal end of the humerus. The head of the humerus fits in the glenoid fossa to complete the shoulder joint. Hence the head is located proximally on the medial aspect of the humerus. The head is palpated when the shoulder joint is laterally rotated.

   Surgical neck: The slightly constricted area just distal to the tubercles where the head meets the body of the humerus.

   Anatomical neck: A circumferential groove separating the head from the tubercles.

   Shaft: Extends from the surgical neck proximally to the epicondyles distally. It is also known as the body of the humerus.

   Greater tubercle: The large projection on the proximal lateral end of the humerus superior to the anatomical neck. Palpate the greater tubercle on your partner by finding the tip of the acromion process and sliding distally onto the greater tubercle of the humerus. You can also place your fingers on the proximal anterior surface of the humerus and medially rotate the humerus, which causes the greater tubercle to move under your fingers.

   Lesser tubercle: A smaller projection on the proximal anterior surface of the humerus medial to the greater tubercle. Palpate the lesser tubercle on your partner by placing your fingers on the proximal anterior surface of the humerus medial to the greater tubercle. Lateral rotation causes the lesser tubercle to move under your fingers.

   Deltoid tuberosity: Located laterally at the midpoint of the shaft of the humerus. The deltoid muscle inserts on the deltoid tuberosity. It is not a well-defined structure, and it is not easily palpated.

   Bicipital groove: Located between the tubercles on the proximal anterior surface of the humerus. It is also called the intertubercular groove. To palpate the bicipital groove on your classmate, place your fingers on the proximal anterior surface of the humerus. Medial and lateral rotation causes the greater and lesser tubercles to move under your fingers. The space between is the bicipital groove. The biceps tendon lies in the bicipital groove. Palpation of the groove may produce discomfort when too much pressure is applied.

4. Locate the following on the skeleton, anatomical models, and at least one partner:

   A. Locate the origin and insertion of the muscle on the skeleton.

   B. Stretch a large rubber band taut by placing one end at the origin and the other end at the insertion of the muscle on the skeleton.

   C. Perform the motion that the muscle does and observe how the rubber band becomes less taut and shorter, similar to the muscle shortening as it contracts.

   D. Perform the opposite motion and observe how the rubber band becomes more taut and longer, similar to the muscle lengthening as it is being stretched.

E. After locating the muscle on the skeleton, locate the muscle on your partner. The position described for locating the muscle on your partner is the manual muscle test position for a fair or better grade of muscle strength. Not all origins, insertions, and muscle bellies can be palpated on your partner.

F. When possible, palpate the origin, insertion, and muscle belly of each muscle by:

1) Placing your fingers on the origin and insertion and asking your partner to contract the muscle.

2) Moving your fingers from the origin to the insertion over the contracting muscle.

3) Asking your partner to relax the muscle and again moving your fingers from the origin to the insertion over the muscle.

SITTING POSITION

Anterior deltoid: Located superficially and anterior to the shoulder joint.

Position:	Sit facing the examiner with the arm relaxed at the side.
Origin:	Lateral third of the clavicle.
Insertion:	Deltoid tuberosity.
Action:	Flex the shoulder to 90 degrees with the elbow extended or flexed.
Palpate:	Approximately 2 inches distal to the lateral clavicle.

Middle deltoid: Located superficially and superior to the shoulder joint.

Position:	Sit facing the examiner with the arm relaxed at the side.
Origin:	Acromion process.
Insertion:	Deltoid tuberosity.
Action:	Abduct the shoulder to 90 degrees with the elbow either extended or flexed to 90 degrees.
Palpate:	Approximately 2 inches distal to the acromion process on the lateral aspect of the humerus.

Supraspinatus: Located deep to the upper trapezius.

Position:	Sit facing away from the examiner with the arm relaxed at the side.
Origin:	Supraspinous fossa of the scapula.
Insertion:	Greater tubercle of the humerus.
Action:	Abduct the shoulder to 90 degrees with the elbow extended or flexed.
Palpate:	This muscle is difficult to palpate because it is deep to the upper trapezius. The muscle belly is superior to the spine of the scapula.

Coracobrachialis: Located deep to the anterior deltoid and the pectoralis major, and anterior to the shoulder joint. It cannot be palpated easily.

Position:	Sit facing the examiner with the arm relaxed at the side.
Origin:	Coracoid process of the scapula.
Insertion:	Medial surface of the humerus near the midpoint of the shaft.
Action:	Flex the shoulder to 90 degrees with the elbow extended.
Palpate:	This muscle is difficult to palpate because it is deep to other shoulder muscles. An alternative method is to place the hand on the hip and, while the person isometrically adducts the shoulder joint, to palpate on the anterior medial surface of the proximal humerus.

PRONE POSITION

Posterior deltoid: Located superficially and posterior to the shoulder joint.

Position:	Lie prone with the shoulder abducted to 90 degrees and the elbow flexed over the edge of the table.
Origin:	Spine of the scapula.
Insertion:	Deltoid tuberosity.
Action:	Lift the arm off the table by performing shoulder horizontal abduction.
Palpate:	Approximately 2 inches distal to the acromion process on the posterior surface of the shoulder joint.

Latissimus dorsi: Located superficially on the posterior thorax.

Position:	Lie prone with the arm medially rotated at the side.
Origin:	Spinous process of T7–L5, posterior surface of the sacrum, iliac crest, and lower three ribs.
Insertion:	Medial lip of the bicipital groove of the humerus.
Action:	Reach across the back toward the opposite hip.
Palpate:	On the side of the thorax near the axilla.

Teres major: Located superficially on the posterior thorax.

Position:	Lie prone with the arm medially rotated at the side.
Origin:	Axillary border of the scapula near the inferior angle.
Insertion:	Crest of the humerus just inferior to the lesser tubercle and next to the insertion of the latissimus dorsi muscle.
Action:	Reach across the back toward the opposite hip.
Palpate:	On the lateral border of the scapula below the axilla. Alternative method: In the prone position, abduct the shoulder joint to 90 degrees with the elbow flexed over the edge of the table so that the forearm is off the table and pronated. Medially rotate the shoulder joint by raising the palm of the hand toward the ceiling. Palpate the muscle belly lateral and superior to the inferior angle of the scapula.

Infraspinatus: Located on the scapula deep to the middle and lower trapezius.

Position:	Lie prone with the shoulder at 90 degrees of abduction and the elbow flexed over the edge of the table.
Origin:	Infraspinous fossa of scapula.
Insertion:	Greater tubercle of the humerus.
Action:	Raise the back of the hand toward the ceiling, producing shoulder lateral rotation.
Palpate:	Over the infraspinous fossa below the spine of the scapula.

Teres minor: Located on the posterior thorax partially deep to the middle and lower trapezius.

Position:	Lie prone with the shoulder at 90 degrees of abduction and the elbow flexed over the edge of the table.
Origin:	Axillary border of the scapula.
Insertion:	Greater tubercle of the humerus.
Action:	Raise the back of the hand toward the ceiling, producing shoulder lateral rotation.

Palpate: Along the axillary border of the scapula.

SUPINE POSITION

Subscapularis: Located deep in the axilla.

     Position: Lie supine with the arm at the side and the elbow flexed to 90 degrees.

     Origin: Subscapular fossa of the scapula.

     Insertion: Lesser tubercle of the humerus.

     Action: Resist shoulder medial rotation (placing the forearm across the abdomen).

     Palpate: At the insertion, or in the axilla anterior to the latissimus dorsi.

Pectoralis major—clavicular portion: Located superficially on the anterior thorax.

     Position: Lie supine with the shoulder in 60 degrees of abduction.

     Origin: Medial one-third of the clavicle.

     Insertion: Lateral lip of the bicipital groove of the humerus.

     Action: Horizontally adduct and flex the shoulder.

     Palpate: Just below the medial one-third of the clavicle.

Pectoralis major—sternal portion: Located superficially on the anterior thorax.

     Position: Lie supine with the shoulder in 120 degrees of abduction.

     Origin: Sternum and costal cartilage of the first six ribs.

     Insertion: Lateral lip of the bicipital groove of the humerus.

     Action: Extend and adduct toward the opposite hip.

     Palpate: At the origin or at the lower anterior border of the axilla.

5. Use a disarticulated skeleton or anatomical model of the shoulder joint and apply the rules of joint arthokinematics and the concave-convex rule to perform the following exercises.

     A. Underline the correct answer.

        The head of the humerus is: concave   convex.

        The glenoid fossa is: concave   convex.

     B. Move the distal bone, the humerus, on the proximal bone, the glenoid fossa of the scapula in all planes of motion. This is an open kinetic chain activity.

     C. Observe the movement of the head of the humerus on the glenoid fossa. Circle the motions that you observed.

        Spin   Roll   Glide   None

     D. Observe the movement of the distal end of the humerus in relation to the movement of the proximal end of the humerus as you move the head of the humerus on the glenoid fossa. Does the distal end of the humerus move in the same direction as or in the opposite direction of the proximal end of the humerus?_____

     E. List the muscles that assist the head of the humerus to move in the glenoid fossa without impingement against the acromion._____

6. **A.** When holding a backpack in one hand with the elbow extended, the force acting on the shoulder joint is:

   Approximation   Traction

   B. Name the muscles acting at the shoulder joint to counteract the force produced by the

   backpack: _____

   _____

   _____

   C. Name the muscles acting at the shoulder girdle to counteract the force produced by the

   backpack: _____

   _____

7. A patient with zero strength of the elbow extensors can extend the elbow using the pectoralis major muscle. Assume and describe the position in which the pectoralis major becomes an elbow extensor.

   _____

   _____

   _____

8. Analyze what happens when an individual lying supine in the anatomical position *raises both arms to 180 degrees*, causing the lumbar lordosis to increase.

   A. What joint motion was performed? _____

   B. What muscle is being elongated over more than one joint? _____

   C. Is this an example of active or passive insufficiency? _____

   D. Explain how this causes an increased lumbar lordosis: _____

   _____

9. Diagram the lever that describes *shoulder flexion, from 0 to 90 degrees*, in the supine position.

   A. On the figure, label the Xs that represent the axis, muscle, and gravity, and identify the specific joint and muscle group.

   B. Make arrows out of the vertical lines to indicate the direction of the movement, the direction of the pull of the muscle, and the direction of gravity.

   C. Identify the muscle and gravity as either *force* or *resistance*.

   X   X   X

   Direction of movement

10. Analyze the motion of *shoulder flexion* diagrammed in question 9 by answering the following questions.

    A. Which joint motion is being analyzed? _____

    B. Identify the "axis" of the motion: _____

    C. Is the "force" producing the movement a muscle or gravity? _____

    D. Is the "resistance" to the movement a muscle or gravity? _____

    E. Which major muscle group is the agonist? _____

    F. Which major muscle group is the antagonist? _____

    G. Is the muscle acting to overcome gravity or slow down gravity? _____

    H. Is the agonist performing a concentric or an eccentric contraction? _____

    I. Is this an open or closed kinetic chain activity? _____

11. Diagram the lever that describes *shoulder flexion, from 90 to 180 degrees*, in the supine position.

    A. On the figure, label the Xs that represent the axis, muscle, and gravity, and identify the specific joint and muscle group.

    B. Make arrows out of the vertical lines to indicate the direction of the movement, the direction of the pull of the muscle, and the direction of gravity.

    C. Identify the muscle and gravity as either *force* or *resistance*.

Direction of movement

12. Analyze the motion of *shoulder flexion* diagrammed in question 11 by answering the following questions.

    A. Which joint motion is being analyzed? _____

    B. Identify the "axis" of the motion: _____

    C. Is the "force" producing the movement a muscle or gravity? _____

    D. Is the "resistance" to the movement a muscle or gravity? _____

    E. Which major muscle group is the agonist? _____

    F. Which major muscle group is the antagonist? _____

    G. Is the muscle acting to overcome gravity or slow down gravity? _____

    H. Is the agonist performing a concentric or an eccentric contraction? _____

    I. Is the antagonist contracting? _____

    J. Is this an open or closed kinetic chain activity? _____

13. Diagram the lever that describes *shoulder extension, from 180 to 90 degrees of flexion,* in the supine position.

   A. On the figure, label the Xs that represent the axis, muscle, and gravity, and identify the specific joint and muscle group.

   B. Make arrows out of the vertical lines to indicate the direction of the movement, the direction of the pull of the muscle, and the direction of gravity.

   C. Identify the muscle and gravity as either *force* or *resistance*.

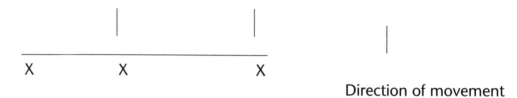

Direction of movement

14. Analyze the motion of *shoulder extension* diagrammed in question 13 by answering the following questions.

   A. Which joint motion is being analyzed? _____

   B. Identify the "axis" of the motion: _____

   C. Is the "force" producing the movement a muscle or gravity? _____

   D. Is the "resistance" to the movement a muscle or gravity? _____

   E. Which major muscle group is the agonist? _____

   F. Which major muscle group is the antagonist? _____

   G. Is the muscle acting to overcome gravity or slow down gravity? _____

   H. Is the agonist performing a concentric or an eccentric contraction? _____

   I. Is this an open or closed kinetic chain activity? _____

15. Diagram the lever that describes *shoulder extension from 90 to 0 degrees,* in the supine position.

   A. On the figure, label the Xs that represent the axis, muscle, and gravity, and identify the specific joint and muscle group.

   B. Make arrows out of the vertical lines to indicate the direction of the movement, the direction of the pull of the muscle, and the direction of gravity.

   C. Identify the muscle and gravity as either *force* or *resistance*.

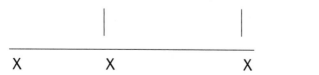

Direction of movement

16. Analyze the motion of *shoulder extension* diagrammed in question 15 by answering the following questions.

    A. Which joint motion is being analyzed? _____

    B. Identify the "axis" of the motion: _____

    C. Is the "force" producing the movement a muscle or gravity? _____

    D. Is the "resistance" to the movement a muscle or gravity? _____

    E. Which major muscle group is the agonist? _____

    F. Which major muscle group is the antagonist? _____

    G. Is the muscle acting to overcome gravity or slow down gravity? _____

    H. Is the agonist performing a concentric or an eccentric contraction? _____

    I. Is this an open or closed kinetic chain activity? _____

17. Diagram the lever that describes *shoulder extension from 180 to 0 degrees* in the sitting position while pulling down weights of an overhead pulley.

    A. On the figure, label the Xs that represent the axis, muscle, and gravity, and identify the specific joint and muscle group.

    B. Make arrows out of the vertical lines to indicate the direction of the movement, the direction of the pull of the muscle, and the direction of gravity.

    C. Identify the muscle and gravity as either *force* or *resistance*.

           X   X   X

                                      Direction of movement

18. Analyze the motion of *shoulder extension* diagrammed in question 17 by answering the following questions.

    A. Which joint motion is being analyzed? _____

    B. Is the movement moving with gravity or against gravity? _____

    C. Is there any external force giving resistance to the extremity? _____

    D. Which major muscle group is the agonist? _____

    E. Which major muscle group is the antagonist? _____

    F. Is the agonist performing a concentric or an eccentric contraction? _____

    G. Is this an open or closed kinetic chain activity? _____

POST-LAB QUESTIONS
SHOULDER JOINT

1. When performing shoulder flexion in an open kinetic chain, is the concave surface moving on the convex surface or is the convex surface moving on the concave surface? _____

   _____

   _____

2. List the muscles that attach on the greater tubercle of the humerus.

   _____

   _____

3. List the muscles that cross the shoulder joint posteriorly.

   _____

   _____

4. List the motions of the shoulder joint.

   _____

   _____

5. You are to treat a house painter who fell off a ladder. In addition to sustaining an anterior dislocation of the shoulder, he has axillary nerve damage. Which muscle(s) may be involved?

   _____

6. You are palpating the coracoid process and thinking about the muscles attached to it. List the muscles attaching to the coracoid process. _____

   _____

7. You are palpating the bicipital groove and thinking about the muscles attached on either side.
   A. List the muscle(s) attached to the lateral side of the bicipital groove: _____
   B. List the muscle(s) attached to the medial side of the bicipital groove: _____

   _____

8. A. The teres major and minor muscles attach along the _____ border of the scapula.

   B. The teres _____ muscle is located superior to the teres

   _____ muscle along the scapular border identified in A.

   C. The teres _____ muscle remains on the posterior surface of the shoulder

   while the teres _____ muscle crosses to the anterior surface.

   D. The _____ muscle, running vertically, passes between the teres major and minor in the axilla.

9. The rotator cuff muscles insert deep to the _____ muscle.

10. The _____ and the _____ muscles are responsible for shoulder hyperextension.

11. The _____ muscle is inferior to the supraspinatus muscle, superior to the teres minor and, in part, deep to the trapezius and deltoid muscles.

12. While palpating the borders of the axillae, you are thinking that the anterior border is formed

   by the _____ muscle and the posterior border is formed by the

   _____ muscle.

13. While palpating the acromion process, you are thinking that the _____ muscle passes inferior to the acromion process.

14. The nerve that innervates the deltoid muscle is often injured when the shoulder dislocates.

   A. Identify the nerve. _____

   B. Describe the sensory area innervated by this nerve. _____

   _____

6

ELBOW JOINT

Student's Name _____   Date Due _____

WORKSHEETS

Complete the following questions prior to lab class.

1. On the drawings, label the bones and major landmarks indicated.

HUMERUS	Trochlea	Shaft
	Head	Lateral supracondylar ridge
	Surgical neck	Medial epicondyle
	Olecranon fossa	Lateral epicondyle
	Bicipital groove	Greater tubercle
	Capitulum	Lesser tubercle

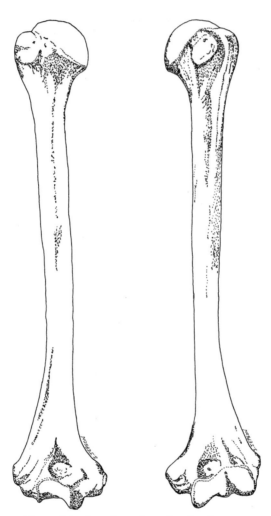

Figure 6.1 *Posterior and anterior view, humerus.*

ULNA Olecranon process   Ulnar tuberosity
Radial notch   Coronoid process
Trochlear notch   Styloid process

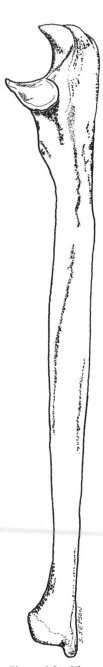

Figure 6.2 Ulna.

RADIUS   Head   Radial tuberosity   Styloid process

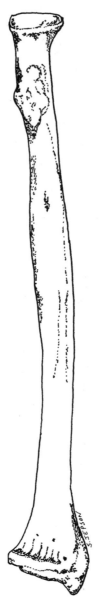

Figure 6.3   *Radius.*

2. On the following drawings,

   A. Label the joints and bones.

   B. Draw the major ligaments indicated.

Humerus	Elbow joint	Lateral collateral ligament
Radius	Proximal radial ulnar joint	Medial collateral ligament
Ulna		

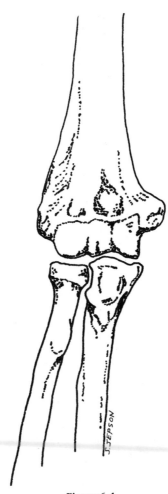

Figure 6.4

Radius   Distal radial ulnar joint   Interosseous membrane
Ulna   Proximal radial ulnar joint   Annular ligament

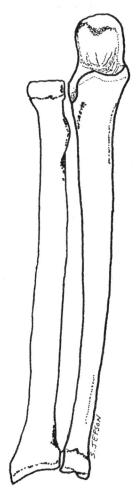

Figure 6.5   *Radius and ulna.*

3. On the drawings,

   A. Label the origin and insertion of the muscles listed.
      Color the origin in red and the insertion in blue.

   B. Join the origin and insertion to show the muscle belly.

   Biceps brachii

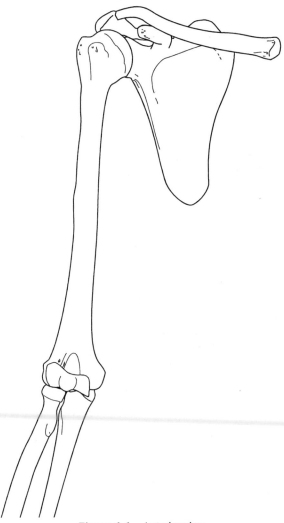

Figure 6.6 *Anterior view.*

Triceps brachii

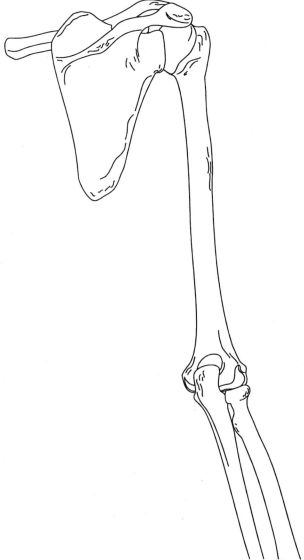

Figure 6.7 *Posterior view.*

Brachialis

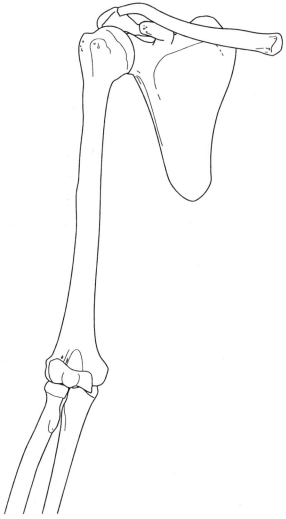

Figure 6.8 *Anterior view.*

Brachioradialis

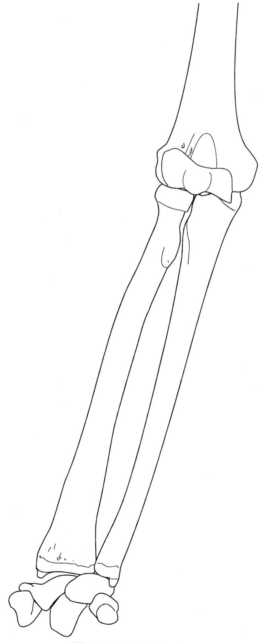

Figure 6.9 *Anterior view.*

Pronator teres   Pronator quadratus

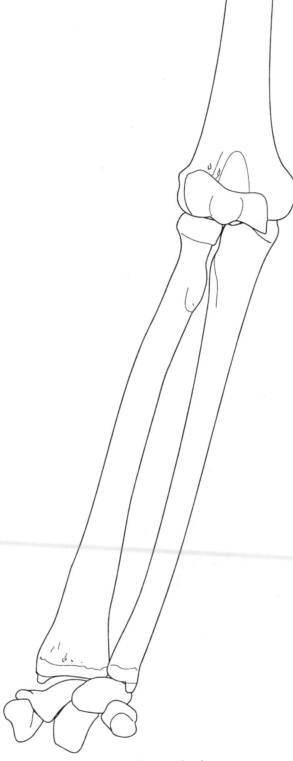

Figure 6.10   *Anterior view.*

Supinator

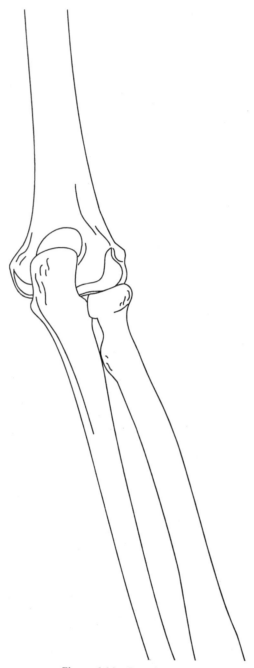

Figure 6.11 *Posterior view.*

Anconeus

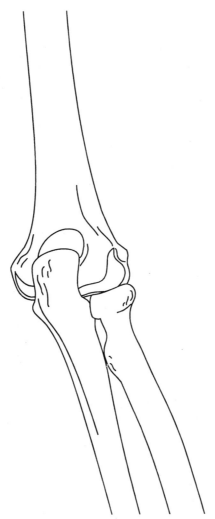

Figure 6.12 *Posterior view.*

4. Identify the characteristics of each joint listed.

Joint	Shape	Number of Axes
ELBOW		
PROXIMAL RADIOULNAR		
DISTAL RADIOULNAR		

5. Indicate which joint structures are concave and which are convex.

Joint	Concave	Convex
ELBOW		
PROXIMAL RADIOULNAR		
DISTAL RADIOULNAR		

6. Match each ligament and structure to the appropriate function or characteristic. Some answers may be used more than once. Some functions or characteristics may have more than one answer.

_____ Attaches to humeral epicondyle and lateral side of ulna

_____ Is triangular in shape

_____ Is ring shaped

_____ Keeps lateral side of joint from separating when stressed

_____ Keeps medial side of joint from separating when stressed

_____ Keeps radius and ulna in contact

_____ Strengthens joint capsule

_____ Attaches to humerus, radius, and ulna

A. Medial collateral ligament
B. Lateral collateral ligament
C. Annular ligament
D. Interosseus membrane
E. Joint capsule

7. For the elbow joint and the forearm joints, indicate which motions are available, in which plane the motion occurs, and the axis of the motion.

Joint	Motions	Plane	Axis
ELBOW			
PROXIMAL RADIOULNAR			
DISTAL RADIOULNAR			

8. For each motion listed, check the muscle(s) that are the major contributors to the motion.

Motion	Brachialis	Brachio-radialis	Biceps Brachii	Supinator	Triceps Brachii	Anconeus	Pronator Teres	Pronator Quadratus
FLEXION								
EXTENSION								
SUPINATION								
PRONATION								

9. For the following multijoint muscles describe each joint position that:

   A. *Lengthens the biceps brachii* muscle simultaneously over all the joints it crosses:_____

   _____

   B. *Lengthens the triceps brachii* muscle simultaneously over all the joints it crosses: _____

   _____

10. Diagram the lever that describes the activity occurring at the *elbow joint when a glass is lowered* to the table.

    A. On the figure, label the Xs that represent the axis, muscle, and gravity, and identify the specific joint and muscle group.

    B. Make arrows out of the vertical lines to indicate the direction of the movement, the direction of the pull of the muscle, and the direction of gravity.

    C. Identify the muscle and gravity as either *force* or *resistance*.

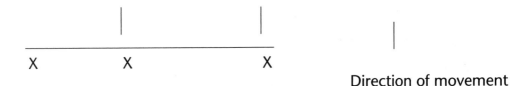

$$\quad$$

X   X   X

Direction of movement

11. Analyze the activity of *lowering a glass* to the table diagrammed in question 10 by answering the following questions:

    A. Which joint motion is being analyzed?_____

    B. Is the movement moving with gravity or against gravity? _____

    C. Is there any external force giving resistance to the extremity? _____

    D. Which major muscle group is the agonist?_____

    E. Which major muscle group is the antagonist?_____

    F. Is the agonist performing a concentric or an eccentric contraction? _____

    G. Is this an open or closed kinetic chain activity? _____

LAB ACTIVITIES
ELBOW JOINT

1. For elbow flexion/extension, and then for forearm supination/pronation:

   A. Place your open left hand in the correct orientation to represent each plane of the motion.

   B. Place your right index finger to indicate the axis of that plane of motion.

2. For each of the joint motions listed below, estimate the degrees of motion available by checking the box that most closely describes that motion (do not use a goniometer). The starting position for the elbow is the anatomical position. The starting position for the radioulnar joint is the fundamental position (also called midposition) with the elbow flexed 90 degrees and the thumb pointing toward the ceiling.

Joints and Motions	0–45	46–90	91–135	136–180
ELBOW				
FLEXION				
EXTENSION				
RADIOULNAR				
SUPINATION				
PRONATION				

3. The carrying angle is measured as the medial angle of the elbow with the upper extremity in the anatomical position. The axis of the goniometer is placed anterior to the elbow joint. One arm of the goniometer is aligned over the long axis of the humerus and the other arm of the goniometer is aligned over the long axis of the forearm.

   A. Measure the carrying angle of four of your classmates. Measure two women and two men, if possible.

Men	Women
1)	1)
2)	2)

   B. What are considered the normal ranges?

   _____

   C. How do these measurements compare to the normal ranges?

   _____

   D. Describe the bony structure alignment that creates the carrying angle.

   _____

   _____

4. On the skeleton, anatomical models, and at least one partner, locate, palpate, and observe the structures listed below. The reference position is the anatomical position. Having pictures for reference is helpful when trying to find structures. Not all structures can be palpated on your partner.

Humerus

Trochlea: Located at the distal medial aspect of the humerus. The trochlea articulates with the ulna. Because this structure is within the elbow joint, it cannot be palpated.

Capitulum: Located on the distal lateral aspect of the humerus. The capitulum articulates with the head of the radius. Because this structure is within the elbow joint, it cannot be palpated.

Medial epicondyle: Located proximal to the trochlea on the medial aspect of the distal end of the humerus. This is the bony protuberance that can be observed and palpated on the medial aspect of the elbow.

Lateral epicondyle: Located proximal to the capitulum on the lateral aspect of the distal end of the humerus. This is the bony protuberance that can be observed and palpated on the lateral aspect of the elbow.

Olecranon fossa: Located on the posterior surface of the distal humerus between the medial and lateral epicondyles. Because it is deep to the triceps, it can be difficult to palpate. Flexing the elbow to about 90 degrees moves the olecranon out of the fossa without significantly stretching the triceps (causing it to become taut) and hence may allow palpation of the olecranon fossa.

Lateral supracondylar ridge: Extends proximally from the lateral epicondyle for 1 to 3 inches. It is palpable as a ridge or edge.

Ulna

Olecranon process: The hook-shaped protuberance located at the proximal end of the ulna. This is the large bump located on the posterior side of the flexed elbow. With your fingers on the olecranon process, have your partner flex and extend an elbow. Feel the olecranon process's shape and movement.

Trochlear notch: Located on the anterior surface of the olecranon process of the ulna. It is also called the **semilunar notch**. The trochlear notch articulates with the trochlea of the humerus. Because this structure is within the elbow joint, it cannot be palpated.

Radial notch: Located just distal to the trochlear notch on the lateral aspect of the ulna. This is where the head of the radius articulates with the ulna. Because this structure is within the joint, it cannot be palpated.

Styloid process: The projection located posteriorly and medially on the distal end of the ulna. This is the bump located medially on the posterior distal surface of the forearm at the wrist.

Coranoid process: Located just below the trochlear notch. With the ulnar tuberosity, it provides attachment for the brachialis muscle. Because it lies deep to muscles, it cannot be palpated.

Ulnar tuberosity: Located below the coranoid process. It provides an attachment for the brachialis muscle. Because it lies deep to muscles, it cannot be palpated.

Radius

Head: The rounded proximal end of the radius. To palpate the head of the radius, hold your partner's forearm flexed at the elbow. Place the fingers of your other hand on the lateral aspect of the forearm just distal to the elbow joint. You should feel the head of the radius move under your fingers as you pronate and supinate the forearm.

Radial tuberosity: Located distal to the head and on the medial aspect of the radius. Because this structure is deep to muscles, it cannot be palpated easily.

Styloid process: The protuberance at the posterior lateral aspect of the distal radius. The radial styloid process is not as prominent as the ulnar styloid process. The radial styloid process is palpated at the lateral aspect of the wrist.

5. On the skeleton, anatomical models, and at least one partner, locate the muscles listed below.

   A. Locate the origin and insertion of the muscle on the skeleton.

   B. Stretch a large rubber band taut by placing one end at the origin and the other end at the insertion of the muscle on the skeleton.

   C. Perform the motion that the muscle does and observe how the rubber band becomes less taut and shorter, similar to the muscle shortening as it contracts.

   D. Perform the opposite motion and observe how the rubber band becomes more taut and longer, similar to the muscle lengthening as it is being stretched.

   E. After locating the muscle on the skeleton, locate the muscle on your partner. The position described for locating the muscle is the manual muscle test position for a fair or better grade of muscle strength. Not all origins, insertions, and muscle bellies can be palpated on your partner.

   F. When possible, palpate the origin, insertion, and muscle belly of each muscle by:

      1) Placing your fingers on the origin and insertion and asking your partner to contract the muscle.

      2) Moving your fingers from the origin to the insertion over the contracting muscle.

      3) Asking your partner to relax the muscle and again moving your fingers from the origin to the insertion over the muscle.

SITTING POSITION

Brachialis: Located on the anterior surface of the arm deep to the biceps brachii.

   Position: Sit facing the examiner with the arm at the side and the forearm pronated.

   Origin: Anterior surface of the distal half of the humerus.

   Insertion: Coronoid process and ulnar tuberosity.

   Action: Flex the elbow. Separating the action of the three elbow flexors is difficult.

   Palpate: Place your fingers on either side of the biceps at the distal end of the humerus.

Brachioradialis: Located superficially on the lateral side of the forearm.

   Position: Sit facing the examiner with the arm at the side and the forearm in mid-position, halfway between supination and pronation.

   Origin: Lateral supracondylar ridge of the humerus.

   Insertion: Distal lateral aspect of the radius just proximal to the radial styloid process.

   Action: Flex the elbow.

   Palpate: Just distal to the elbow joint on the lateral side over the muscle belly.

Biceps brachii: Located superficially on the anterior aspect of the humerus.

   Position: Sit facing the examiner with the arm at the side and the forearm supinated.

   Origin: Long head: supraglenoid tubercle of the scapula.
   Short head: coracoid process of the scapula.

   Insertion: Radial tuberosity.

   Action: Flex the elbow.

   Palpate: The origins of the long head of the biceps cannot be palpated. Near its origin, the short head of the biceps tendon can be palpated in the bicipital groove. The insertion of the biceps tendon on the radius is palpated easily when the muscle contracts. The muscle belly is superficial and easily palpated on the anterior surface of the middle and distal humerus.

Supinator: Located deep on the lateral aspect of the elbow.

Position: Sit facing the examiner with the arm at the side and the forearm in the midposition.

Origin: Lateral epicondyle of the humerus and posterior lateral aspect of the adjacent ulna.

Insertion: Anterior surface of the proximal radius.

Action: Supinate the forearm.

Palpate: On the lateral aspect of the elbow.

Pronator teres: Located superficially on the medial aspect of the elbow.

Position: Sit with the arm at the side, the elbow flexed to 90 degrees, and the forearm in midposition.

Origin: Medial epicondyle of the humerus and coronoid process of ulna.

Insertion: Lateral aspect of the radius at the midpoint of the shaft.

Action: Pronate the forearm—turn the palm toward the floor.

Palpate: On the anterior surface of the proximal one-third of the forearm between the origin and insertion. Resisting the pronation may make the muscle easier to find.

Pronator quadratus: Located deep on the anterior distal surface of the forearm.

Position: Sit with the arm at the side, the elbow flexed to 90 degrees, and the forearm in the midposition.

Origin: Anterior surface of the distal one-fourth of the ulna.

Insertion: Anterior surface of the distal one-fourth of the radius.

Action: Pronate the forearm.

Palpate: The pronator quadratus may be difficult to palpate because it is deep to many tendons of the wrist and hand muscles.

PRONE POSITION

Triceps brachii: Located superficially on the posterior surface of the humerus.

Position: Lie prone with the shoulder abducted to 90 degrees and the elbow flexed over the edge of the table.

Origin: Long head: Infraglenoid tubercle of the scapula.
Lateral head: Inferior to the greater tubercle on the posterior side of the humerus.
Medial head: Posterior surface of the humerus.

Insertion: Olecranon process of the ulna.

Action: Minimally assist with elbow extension.

Palpate: On the posterior surface of the humerus.

Anconeus: Located superficially on the posterior aspect of the elbow.

Position: Lie prone with the shoulder abducted to 90 degrees and the elbow flexed over the edge of the table.

Origin: Lateral epicondyle of the humerus.

Insertion: Lateral and inferior to the triceps on the olecranon process of the ulna.

Action: Minimally assist with elbow extension.

Palpate: This small muscle is not present in all individuals and is difficult to separate accurately from the triceps.

6. For the following activities about multijoint muscles, refer to question 9 in the worksheets.

   A. Assume the joint positions that shorten the biceps brachii over all the joints it crosses. What is the effect on the triceps? _____

   B. Assume the joint positions that lengthen the biceps brachii over all the joints it crosses. What is the effect on the triceps? _____

7. Using the skeleton or a model of the elbow joint, and applying the rules of joint arthokinematics and the concave-convex rule,

   A. Move the *distal bones (radius and ulna)* of the elbow joint on the proximal bone (humerus) as would occur in an open kinetic chain activity.

   B. Underline the correct answer.

   The distal end of the humerus is: concave   convex.

   The proximal end of the radius is: concave   convex.

   The proximal end of the ulna is: concave   convex.

   C. Observe the movement of the *proximal ends of the radius and ulna* on the humerus during an open kinetic chain activity. Circle the motions that you observe.

   Spin   Roll   Glide   None

   D. Observe the movement of the *distal ends of the radius and ulna* during a open kinetic chain activity. Does the distal end move in the same direction or in the opposite direction as the proximal ends of the bones during elbow movement? _____

   E. Move the *proximal bone (humerus)* of the elbow joint on the distal bones (radius and ulna) as would occur in a closed kinetic chain activity.

   F. Observe the movement of the *distal end of the humerus* on the radius and ulna during a closed kinetic chain activity. Circle the motions that you observe.

   Spin   Roll   Glide   None

   G. Observe the movement of the *proximal end of the humerus*. Does the distal end move in the same direction or in the opposite direction as the proximal end of the humerus during movement at the elbow joint in a closed kinetic chain activity? _____

   _____

8. The strength of a muscle can be tested with the individual in the test position for a fair grade or better muscle strength. To test the strength of the elbow flexors, have your lab partner put his or her elbow in flexion and hold it in that position while you try to move it into extension.

   Test the strength of the *elbow flexors* with the forearm positioned first in pronation, second in supination, and third in midposition.

   A. Did the position of the forearm affect strength of elbow flexion? _____

   B. Explain your answer. _____

   _____

   _____

Test the strength of *elbow extensors* with the forearm positioned first in pronation, second in supination, and third in midposition.

C. Did the position of the forearm affect strength of the triceps? _____

D. Explain your answer. _____

_____

9. Analyze elbow extension in the following activities.

First activity: Perform a push-up from the prone position. Consider the *up phase* of the activity.

Second activity: In the sitting position, perform elbow extension starting with the upper extremity in full shoulder and elbow flexion.

A. Which activity is an example of reversal of muscle action? _____

B. Explain your answer. _____

_____

C. Which activity is an example of an open kinetic chain activity? _____

D. Which activity is an example of a closed kinetic chain activity? _____

E. In the first activity, is traction or approximation occurring at the elbow joint? _____

POST-LAB QUESTIONS
ELBOW JOINT

After completing the Worksheets and Lab Activities, answer the following questions without using your books or notes. When finished, check your answers.

1. Name the ring-shaped ligament within which the radius rotates: _____

2. You are palpating the arm of a patient.

    A. Name the muscle that lies deep to the biceps brachii near the distal end of the humerus.

    _____

    B. Name the muscle that lies deep to the biceps at the shoulder. _____

3. Name the nerve that lies in the groove between the medial epicondyle and the olecranon process.

    _____

4. Match the nerve with the muscle it innervates (answers may be used more than once):

    _____ Biceps brachii   A. Musculocutaneous
                                            B. Radial
    _____ Triceps brachii   C. Median

    _____ Pronator teres

    _____ Supinator

    _____ Brachialis

    _____ Brachioradialis

    _____ Pronator quadratus

5. You are to treat an individual who had a midshaft fracture of the humerus. A complication of this injury was damage to the radial nerve, resulting in paralysis.

    A. Which elbow and/or forearm muscles would have lost innervation? _____

    _____

    B. What motions will the individual have difficulty performing? _____

    _____

6. Identify the bone on which the bony landmarks are located and the muscle(s) that attach there.

Bony Landmark	Bone	Muscle(s)
MEDIAL EPICONDYLE		
LATERAL EPICONDYLE		
LATERAL SUPRACONDYLAR RIDGE		
OLECRANON PROCESS		
CORONOID PROCESS		
ULNAR TUBEROSITY		
RADIAL STYLOID PROCESS		
RADIAL TUBEROSITY		

7. Identify the bones and motions of the joints listed below.

Joint	Bones	Motions
ELBOW		
PROXIMAL RADIOULNAR		
DISTAL RADIOULNAR		

8. Which muscle lies deep to the wrist and finger flexors at the distal forearm? _____

9. Why must a muscle attach on the radius to be able to pronate or supinate the forearm? _____

_____

10. A. Which muscles that cause motion of the elbow joint do not attach to the radius? _____

_____

   B. Do any of these muscles cause pronation or supination? _____

11. When elbow flexion is performed and supination is not desired, what muscle(s) prevents the supination? _____

12. Identify the following nonmuscular structures.

   A. This structure crosses the elbow vertically on the radial side attaching to the humerus and ulna: _____

   B. This structure crosses the elbow vertically on the ulnar side attaching to the humerus and ulna: _____

   C. This structure attaches only to the ulna: _____

   D. This structure connects the ulna and the radius via a broad attachment: _____

_____

13. Analyze the following two activities by answering the questions that follow.

    First activity: An individual pulling on a rope attached to a boat is bringing the boat into the shore.

    Second activity: An individual is climbing up a rope.

    A. In the first activity, which attachment of the elbow flexors is moving toward the other attachment? _____

    B. In the second activity, which attachment of the elbow flexors is moving toward the other attachment? _____

    C. Which activity is an example of the reversal of muscle action? _____

14. When the radial nerve has been severed, has the ability to supinate the forearm been lost? _____
    If not, why? _____

15. When the radial nerve has been severed, has the ability to extend the elbow been lost? _____
    If not, why? _____

16. Is elbow flexion lost when the musculocutaneous nerve has been severed? _____
    If not, why? _____

7

WRIST JOINT

Student's Name _____ Date Due _____

WORKSHEETS

Complete the following questions prior to lab class.

1. On the drawing, label the following joints, bones, and landmarks.

Radius	Trapezium	Radioulnar joint
Ulna	Trapezoid	Midcarpal joint
Scaphoid	Capitate	Carpometacarpal joint
Lunate	Hamate	Ulnar styloid process
Triquetrum	Radial styloid process	Hook of hamate
Pisiform	Radiocarpal joint	Metacarpals 1–5

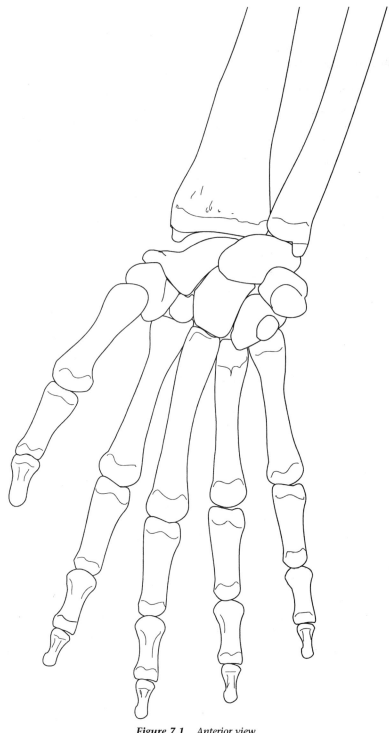

Figure 7.1 *Anterior view.*

2. On the following drawings, draw the major ligaments and structures listed.

Radial collateral ligament   Ulnar collateral ligament   Articular disk

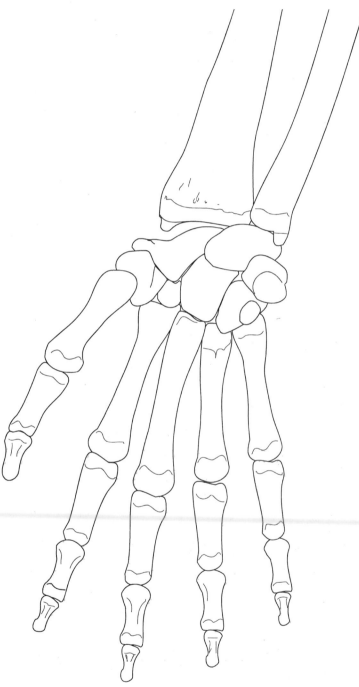

Figure 7.2   *Anterior view.*

Palmar radiocarpal ligament

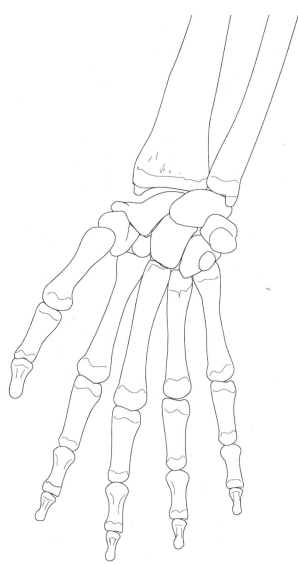

Figure 7.3 *Anterior view.*

Dorsal radiocarpal ligament

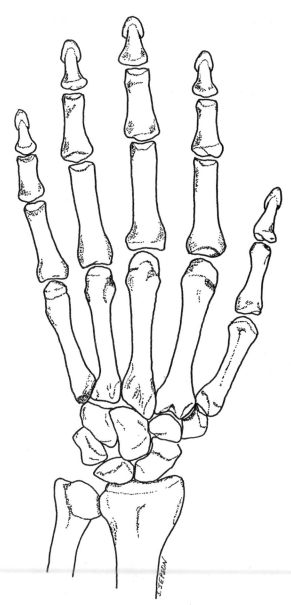

Figure 7.4 *Posterior view.*

Palmar fascia

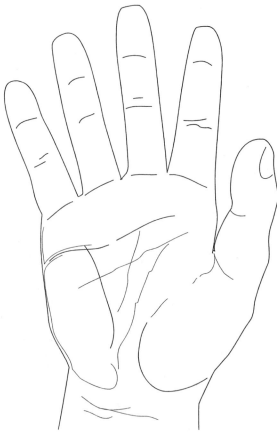

Figure 7.5 *Palmar view.*

3. On the following drawings,

   A. Label the origin and insertion of the muscles listed.
   Color the origin in red and the insertion in blue.

   B. Join the origin and insertion to show the muscle belly.

   Flexor carpi ulnaris

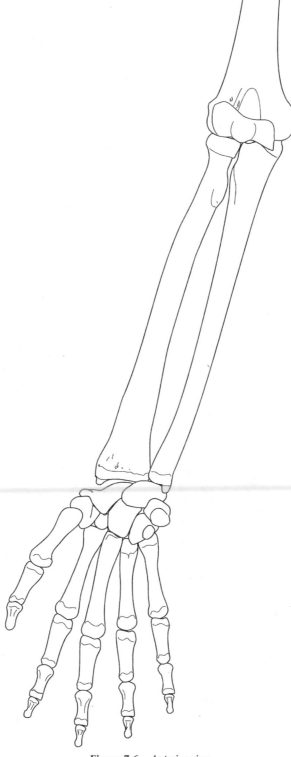

Figure 7.6 Anterior view.

Flexor carpi radialis

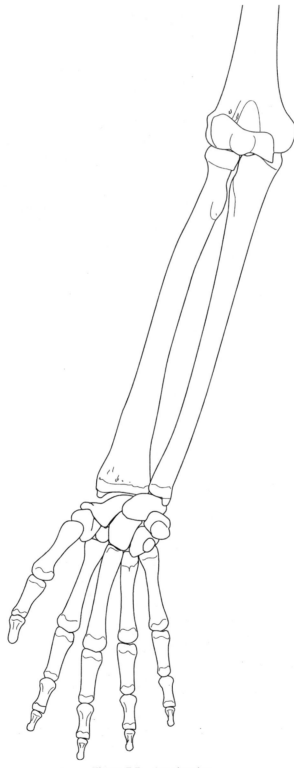

Figure 7.7 *Anterior view.*

Palmaris longus

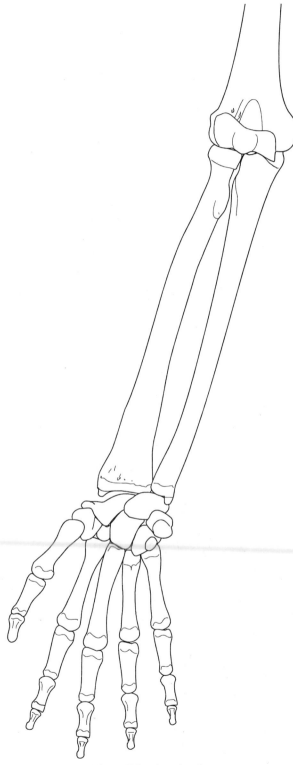

Figure 7.8 *Anterior view.*

Extensor carpi radialis brevis

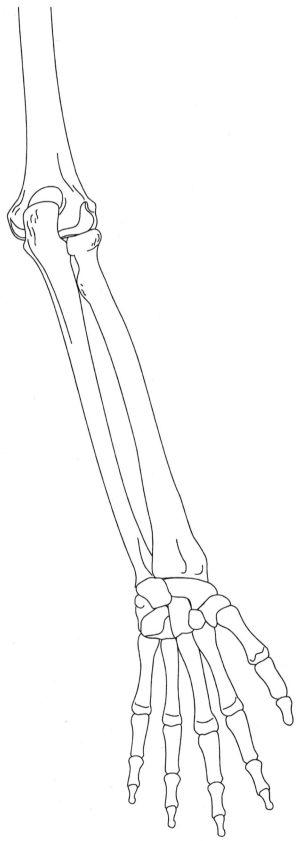

Figure 7.9 *Posterior view.*

Extensor carpi radialis longus

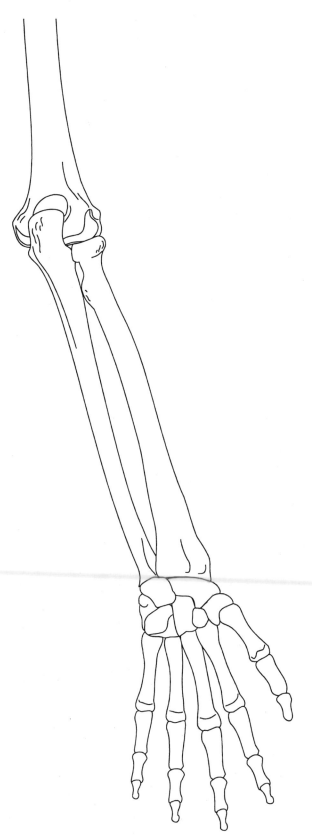

Figure 7.10 *Posterior view.*

Extensor carpi ulnaris

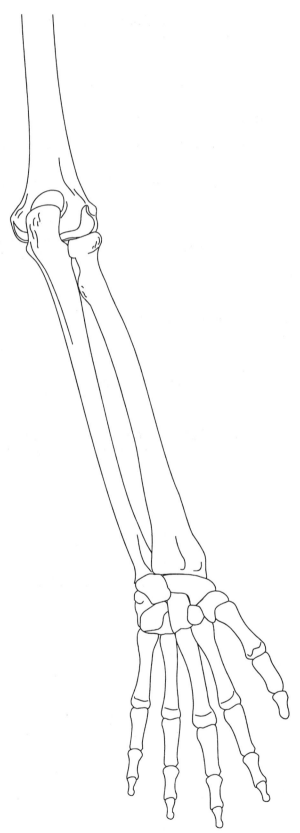

Figure 7.11 *Posterior view.*

4. For each joint listed, identify the following.

Joint	Shape	Number of Planes	Motions
RADIOCARPAL			
MIDCARPAL			

5. Name the structures of the radiocarpal joint that are concave. _____

   Name the structures of the radiocarpal joint that are convex. _____

6. Match each ligament and structure listed below with the appropriate function or characteristic. Use each term only once.

   _____ Limits extension

   _____ Acts as filler between ulna and adjacent carpals

   _____ Provides lateral support

   _____ Limits flexion

   _____ Provides protection and muscle attachment

   _____ Provides medial support

   A. Radial collateral ligament
   B. Ulnar collateral ligament
   C. Palmar radiocarpal ligament
   D. Dorsal radiocarpal ligament
   E. Articular disk
   F. Palmar fascia

7. For each motion listed, check the muscle(s) that perform the motion.

Motion	Flexor carpi ulnaris	Flexor carpi radialis	Extensor carpi radialis longus	Extensor carpi radialis brevis	Extensor carpi ulnaris
FLEXION					
EXTENSION					
RADIAL DEVIATION					
ULNAR DEVIATION					

8. Muscles working together can produce motions that an individual muscle cannot produce when it contracts alone.

A. What motions are produced by contracting the flexor carpi ulnaris? _____

_____

B. What motions are produced by contracting the extensor carpi ulnaris? _____

_____

C. What motions are produced by simultaneously contracting the flexor carpi ulnaris and the

extensor carpi ulnaris? _____

D. What motions are produced by contracting the flexor carpi radialis? _____

_____

E. What motions are produced by contracting the extensor carpi radialis longus? _____

_____

F. What motions are produced by simultaneously contracting the flexor carpi radialis and the

extensor carpi radialis longus? _____

G. The flexor carpi radialis and the extensor carpi radialis longus _____ each

other's flexion/extension component and act as _____ to produce radial

deviation.

LAB ACTIVITIES
WRIST JOINT

1. For each of the motions available at the wrist joint,

   A. Place your open left hand in the orientation to represent the plane of the motion.

   B. Place your right index finger to indicate the axis of that plane of motion.

2. For each of the motions available at the wrist joint, estimate the degrees of motion available by checking the box that most closely describes that motion. (Do not use a goniometer.)

Motions	*0–45*	*46–90*	*91–135*	*136–180*
FLEXION				
EXTENSION				
RADIAL DEVIATION				
ULNAR DEVIATION				

3. On the skeleton, anatomical models, and at least one partner, locate, palpate, and observe the structures described below. The reference position is the anatomical position. Having pictures for reference is helpful when trying to find the structures. Because the carpal bones are difficult to palpate, orient your partner's hand in the same orientation as the figure you are using for reference. Placing the figure alongside your partner's hand may also be helpful.

   NOTE: Not all structures can be easily palpated because they lie deep to many tendons and ligaments. Care must be taken when palpating, especially the capitate and the ligaments of the wrist, so as not to cause pain and delayed soreness.

   Radius

   Styloid process: Projection at the distal end of the radius. Palpate at the distal lateral aspect of the radius. Note that the radial styloid process lies more distal than the ulnar process.

   Ulna

   Styloid process: Projection at the distal end of the ulna. Palpate at the distal posterior aspect of the ulna. Note that the ulnar styloid process is more prominent than the radial styloid process.

   NOTE: Place one finger on the ulnar styloid process and one on the radial styloid process and observe that the ulnar styloid process lies more proximal than the radial styloid process.

   Proximal row of carpal bones

   Scaphoid: Located in the proximal row of carpal bones on the radial side of the wrist just distal to the radial styloid process and in line with the thumb.

   Lunate: Located in the proximal row of carpal bones in line with the middle finger.

   Triquetrum: Located in the proximal row of carpal bones on the ulnar side of the wrist just distal to the ulna and in line with the fourth and fifth fingers. The articular disk lies between the ulna and the triquetrum.

   Pisiform: A small bone that appears to lie on the triquetrum on the anterior surface of the palm in line with the fifth finger. It is palpated on the palmar surface. The pisiform is more prominent than the hook of the hamate and is often confused with the hook of the hamate.

Distal row of carpal bones

Trapezium: Located in the distal row of carpal bones on the radial side. It articulates with the first metacarpal bone (thumb).

Trapezoid: A small bone just medial to the trapezium bone in the distal row of carpal bones. It articulates with the second metacarpal bone.

Capitate: The largest carpal bone of the distal row. It articulates with the third metacarpal and part of the fourth metacarpal bones. Palpate the capitate by moving your thumb proximally along the dorsal surface of the metacarpal bone of the middle finger to an indentation just proximal to the third metacarpal. The capitate lies in this indentation. The capitate can be used as the reference point to locate many of the other carpal bones.

Hamate: Located on the ulnar side of the wrist medial to the capitate and in line with the fourth and fifth metacarpals. You can grasp the hamate between your thumb and first finger on the ulnar side of the hand.

Hook of the hamate: The projection on the palmar surface of the hamate. The hook can be palpated using the tip of your thumb with deep pressure applied just medial to the longitudinal arches at the wrist. Remember, the hamate is in the distal row of carpal bones just lateral to the pisiform bone.

Other structures

Radial collateral ligament: Located on the radial side of the wrist. Attachments are the styloid process of the radius proximally and the scaphoid and trapezium distally. Place the pad of one finger over the lateral aspect of the wrist, move the wrist into ulnar deviation, and feel the ligament become taut.

Ulnar collateral ligament: Located on the ulnar side of the wrist. Attachments are the styloid process of the ulna proximally and the pisiform and triquetrum distally. Place the pad of one finger over the medial aspect of the wrist, move the wrist into radial deviation and feel the ligament become taut.

Palmar radiocarpal ligament: Located on the palmar surface of the wrist deep to the wrist and finger flexor tendons. It is a broad, thick band extending from the anterior surface of the distal radius and ulna to the anterior surface of the scaphoid, lunate, and triquetrum. Extending the wrist makes the palmar radiocarpal ligament taut.

Dorsal radiocarpal ligament: Located on the posterior side of the wrist deep to the wrist and finger extensor tendons. The proximal attachment is the distal radius, and the distal attachment is the scaphoid, lunate, and triquetrum. This ligament is not as thick as the palmar radiocarpal ligament. Wrist flexion makes the dorsal radiocarpal ligament taut.

Articular disk: Located on the ulnar side of the wrist between the ulna proximally and the triquetrum and lunate distally.

Palmar fascia: Also known as the palmar aponeurosis, it is located superficially in the palm of the hand at the midline. The palmaris longus tendon and the flexor retinaculum blend into this fascia.

Radiocarpal joint: The articulation of the distal radius with the scaphoid and lunate.

Midcarpal joint: The articulation between the proximal and distal rows of carpal bones. Although not a true joint, it is often considered as such.

4. On the skeleton, anatomical models, and at least one partner, locate the muscles listed below.

   A. Locate the origin and insertion of the muscle on the skeleton.

   B. Stretch a large rubber band taut by placing one end at the origin and the other end at the insertion of the muscle on the skeleton.

   C. Perform the motion that the muscle does and observe how the rubber band becomes less taut and shorter, similar to the muscle shortening as it contracts.

   D. Perform the opposite motion and observe how the rubber band becomes more taut and longer, similar to the muscle lengthening as it is stretched.

E. After locating the muscle on the skeleton, locate the muscle on your partner. The position described for locating the muscle on your partner is the manual muscle test position for a fair or better grade of muscle strength. Not all origins, insertions, and muscle bellies are palpable on your partner.

F. When possible, palpate the origin, insertion, and muscle belly of each muscle by:

1) Placing your fingers on the origin and insertion and asking your partner to contract the muscle.

2) Moving your fingers from the origin to the insertion over the contracting muscle.

3) Asking your partner to relax the muscle and again moving your fingers from the origin to the insertion over the muscle.

SITTING POSITION

Flexor carpi ulnaris: Located superficially along the ulnar side of the forearm.

Position:	Sit with the forearm supinated and the wrist in the neutral position.
Origin:	Medial epicondyle of the humerus.
Insertion:	Pisiform, hamate, and base of the fifth metacarpal.
Action:	Flex the wrist with ulnar deviation.
Palpate:	The tendon on the anterior ulnar side of the wrist and the muscle belly on the anterior ulnar side of the forearm approximately 2 to 3 inches below the elbow.

Flexor carpi radialis: Located superficially on the anterior forearm.

Position:	Sit with the forearm supinated and the wrist in the neutral position.
Origin:	Medial epicondyle of the humerus.
Insertion:	Base of the second and third metacarpals.
Action:	Flex the wrist with radial deviation.
Palpate:	The tendon on the anterior radial side of the wrist and the muscle belly on the anterior and slightly medial surface of the forearm just proximal to the midpoint between the medial epicondyle and the carpometacarpal joint of the thumb. When an individual has a palmaris longus muscle, the flexor carpi radialis tendon lies lateral to the palmaris longus tendon.

Palmaris longus: Located superficially in the midline of the anterior forearm.

Position:	Sit with the forearm supinated and the wrist in the neutral position.
Origin:	Medial epicondyle of the humerus.
Insertion:	Palmar fascia.
Action:	Flex the wrist.
Palpate:	The tendon in the midline on the anterior side of the wrist medial to the flexor carpi radialis tendon. This muscle is absent in some individuals and others may have only one.

Extensor carpi radialis longus: Located superficially on the posterior radial side of the forearm.

Position:	Sit with the forearm pronated and the wrist in the neutral position.
Origin:	Supracondylar ridge of the humerus.
Insertion:	Base of the second metacarpal.
Action:	Extend the wrist with radial deviation.
Palpate:	The tendon on the dorsal side of the wrist proximal to the insertion on the second metacarpal.

Extensor carpi radialis brevis: Located superficially on the posterior radial side of the forearm.

Position:	Sit with the forearm pronated and the wrist in the neutral position.
Origin:	Lateral epicondyle of the humerus.
Insertion:	Base of the third metacarpal.
Action:	Extend the wrist with radial deviation.
Palpate:	The tendon on the dorsal side of the wrist proximal to the insertion on the third metacarpal.

Extensor carpi ulnaris: Located superficially on the posterior side of the forearm.

Position:	Sit with the forearm pronated and the wrist in the neutral position.
Origin:	Lateral epicondyle of the humerus.
Insertion:	Base of the fifth metacarpal.
Action:	Extend the wrist with ulnar deviation.
Palpate:	The tendon on the dorsal side of the wrist between the ulnar styloid process and the fifth metacarpal.

5. Use a disarticulated skeleton or model of the radial carpal joint, and apply the rules of joint arthrokinematics and the concave-convex rule to perform the following exercises.

A. Move the distal bones (the proximal row of carpals) on the proximal bone (the radius) in all planes of motion. This is an open kinetic chain activity.

B. Observe the movement of the proximal end of the moving bones and circle the motions that you observed.

Spin   Roll   Glide   None

C. Flex and extend the proximal bone (the radius) on the distal bones (the proximal row of carpal bones). This is a closed kinetic chain activity.

D. Observe the movement of the proximal and distal ends of the radius as the wrist moves through flexion and extension. Does the proximal end of the radius move in the same or the opposite direction as the distal end? _____

6. A. Using your *right hand*, open a jar with a screw-on lid. Does your hand move into radial or ulnar deviation as you loosen the lid? _____

B. Replace the lid on the jar using your *right hand*. Does your hand move into radial or ulnar deviation as you tighten the lid? _____

C. Using your *left hand*, open a jar with a screw-on lid. Does your hand move into radial or ulnar deviation as you loosen the lid? _____

D. Replace the lid on the jar using your *left hand*. Does your hand move into radial or ulnar deviation as you tighten the lid? _____

POST-LAB QUESTIONS
WRIST JOINT

After you have completed the Worksheets and Lab Activities, answer the following questions without using your books or notes. When finished, check your answers.

1. The wrist flexors share a common proximal attachment on, or in the area of, the _____
   _____

2. List the muscles that attach on the posterior lateral side of the wrist. _____
   _____

3. Which two muscles attach distally on the base of the fifth metacarpal? _____
   _____

4. Which muscle does not have two attachments on bone and what is its nonbony
   attachment? _____

5. List the muscles that act together to produce ulnar deviation of the wrist. _____
   _____

6. List which muscles play the role of a neutralizer during wrist ulnar deviation and list what motion
   each is neutralizing. _____
   _____

7. Can the position of the elbow joint affect the range of motion of the wrist? _____
   Explain your answer. _____
   _____
   _____

8. Explain why the extensor carpi radialis brevis does not play a major role in wrist radial deviation.
   _____
   _____

9. An individual with a diagnosis of ulnar nerve entrapment has signs of muscle weakness. Which
   wrist muscle(s) would be involved? _____
   _____

10. Loss of radial nerve function results in a condition known as "wrist drop." Explain why.

_____

_____

11. Starting on the anterior medial side and proceeding laterally around the wrist, name the wrist muscles in the order encountered. _____

_____

_____

12. Generally speaking, the wrist flexors and extensors are innervated by which nerves?

    A. Wrist extensors: _____

    B. Wrist flexors: _____

    C. List the exception(s): _____

8

HAND

Student's Name _____   Date Due _____

WORKSHEETS

Complete the following questions prior to lab class.

1. On the following drawings,

   A. Label the bones of the hand.

   BONES

   Radius

   Ulna

Carpals	Trapezium	Hamate	Capitate	Trapezoid
	Scaphoid	Lunate	Triquetrum	Pisiform

Metacarpals	1–5

Phalanges	Proximal	Distal	Middle

   B. Draw the structures indicated.

   OTHER STRUCTURES   Flexor retinaculum
   Palmar carpal ligament
   Transverse carpal ligament

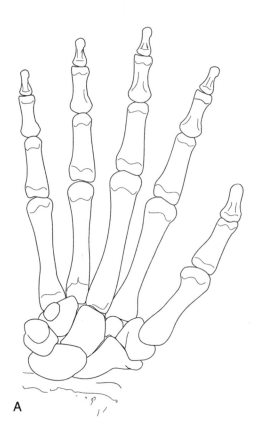

A

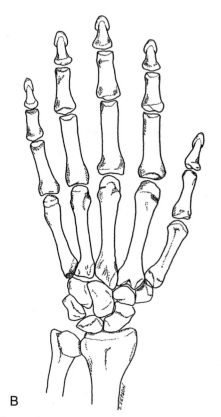

B

Figure 8.1 *(A) Anterior view. (B) Posterior view.*

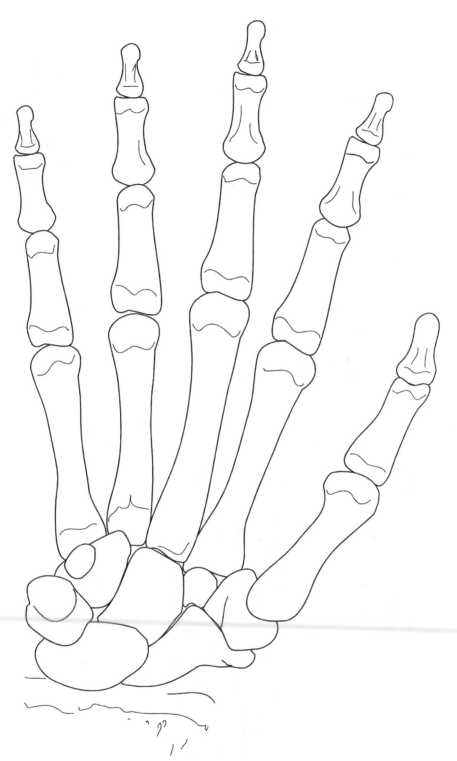

Figure 8.2 *Anterior view.*

2. On the drawing,

   A. Label the joints of the hand.

   JOINTS   Carpometacarpal (CMC)   Proximal interphalangeal (PIP)
                                     Metacarpophalangeal (MP)   Distal interphalangeal (DIP)

   B. Draw the structures indicated.

   OTHER STRUCTURES   Extensor retinaculum   Extensor expansion

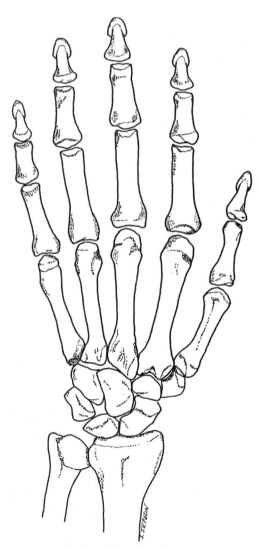

Figure 8.3 *Posterior view.*

3. On the following drawings,

   A. Label the origin and insertion of the muscles listed.
      Color the origin in red and the insertion in blue.

   B. Join the origin and insertion to show the muscle belly.

   Flexor digitorum superficialis   Flexor digitorum profundus

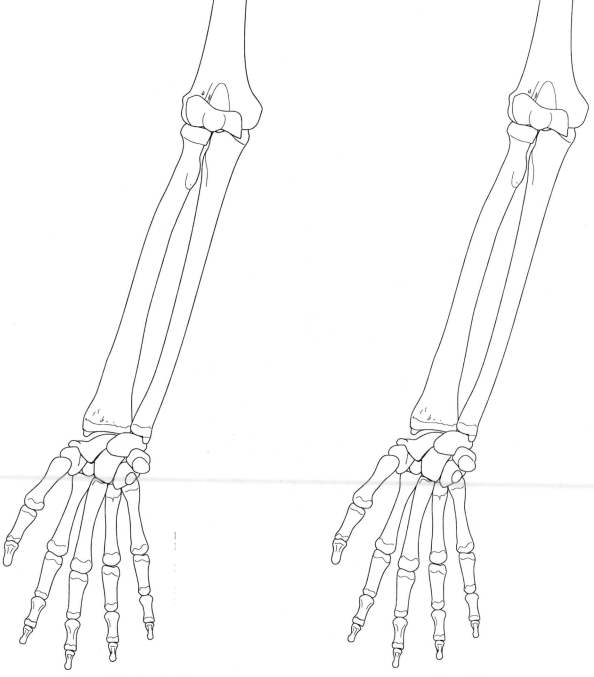

Figure 8.4 *Anterior view.*   **Figure 8.5**

Extensor digitorum

Extensor digiti minimi and extensor indices

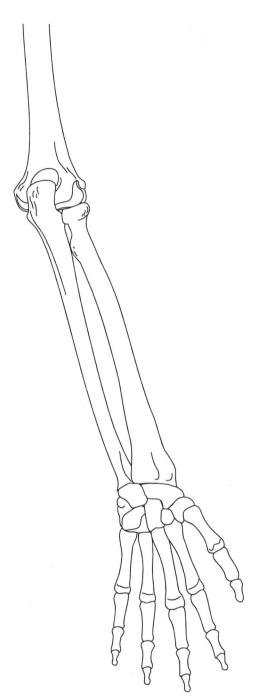

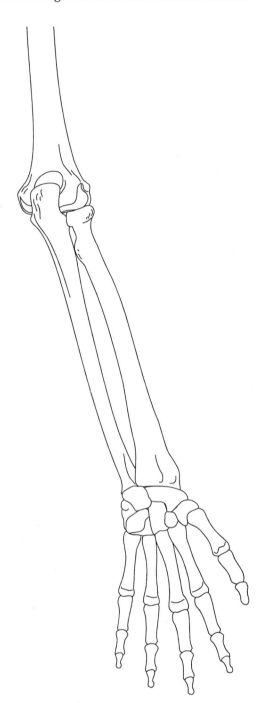

Figure 8.6 *Posterior view.*

Figure 8.7

Flexor pollicis longus

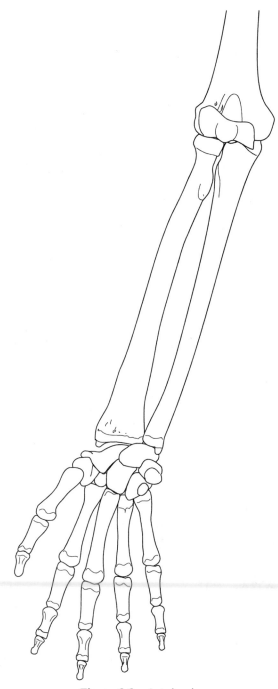

Figure 8.8 *Anterior view.*

Abductor pollicis longus

Extensor pollicis brevis and longus

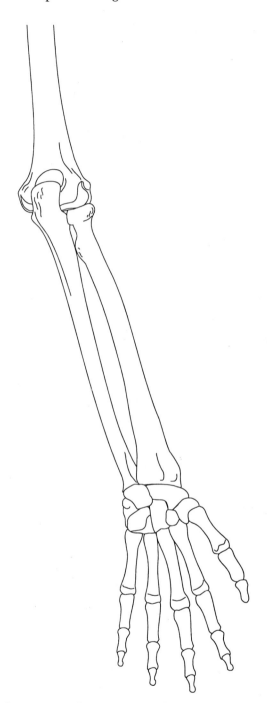

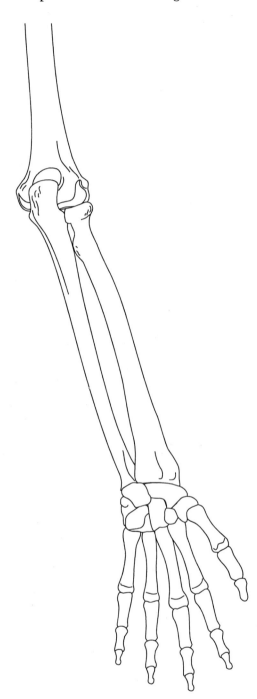

Figure 8.9   *Posterior view.*

Figure 8.10

Flexor pollicis brevis and flexor digiti minimi

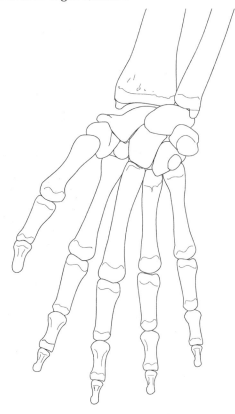

Figure 8.11 *Anterior view.*

Abductor pollicis brevis and abductor digiti minimi

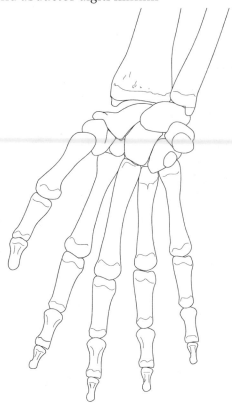

Figure 8.12 *Anterior view.*

Opponens pollicis   Opponens digiti minimi   Adductor pollicis

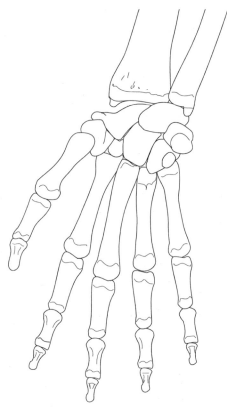

Figure 8.13   *Anterior view.*

Palmar interossei

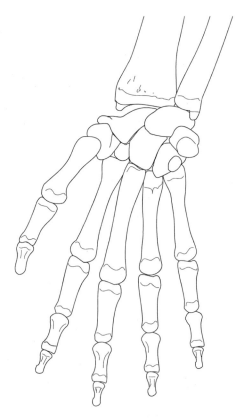

Figure 8.14   *Anterior view.*

Dorsal interossei

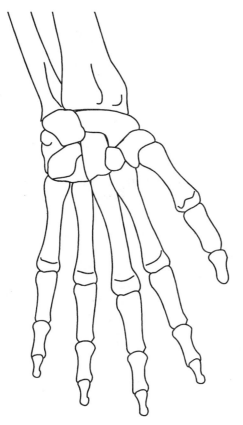

Figure 8.15 *Posterior view.*

4. For each joint listed, identify the following.

Joint	Shape	Number of Axes	Motions
THUMB CMC			
THUMB MP			
THUMB IP			
FINGER MP			
FINGER PIP			
FINGER DIP			

5. Name the concave and convex portions of the following joints.

Joint	Concave	Convex
2ND–5TH MP		
2ND–5TH PIP		
2ND–5TH DIP		

6. Match each ligament and structure listed below with the appropriate function or characteristic. Each term may be used more than once. Each function or characteristic may have more than one answer.

_____ Is located on the anterior surface

_____ Composed of two parts

_____ Is part of carpal tunnel

_____ Holds tendons close to wrist

_____ Is located on posterior surface

_____ Is located on the posterior and sides of the proximal phalanges

_____ Provides attachment of extensor tendons to middle and distal phalanges

A. Flexor retinaculum
B. Extensor retinaculum
C. Extensor expansion
D. Transverse carpal ligament
E. Palmar carpal ligament

7. For each joint listed, indicate which motions are available, in which plane the motion occurs, and the axis of the motion.

Metacarpophalangeal Joints of Fingers 2–5

Motions	Plane	Axis

Carpometacarpal Joint of the Thumb

Motions	Plane	Axis

Proximal and Distal Interphalangeal Joints of Fingers 2–5

Motions	Plane	Axis

8. For each motion listed, check the muscle(s) that are major contributors to that motion.

Motion	Flexor digitorum superficialis	Flexor digitorum profundus	Flexor pollicis longus	Extensor digitorum	Extensor digiti minimi	Extensor indicis	Abductor pollicis longus	Extensor pollicis longus	Extensor pollicis brevis
FLEXION									
EXTENSION									
ABDUCTION									
ADDUCTION									
OPPOSITION									

Motion	Flexor pollicis brevis	Abductor pollicis brevis	Opponens pollicis	Flexor digiti minimi	Abductor digiti minimi	Opponens digiti minimi	Adductor pollicis	Dorsal interossei	Palmar interossei	Lumbricales
FLEXION										
EXTENSION										
ABDUCTION										
ADDUCTION										
OPPOSITION										

9. Of the extrinsic muscles listed in question 8,

   A. List those muscles that are multijoint muscles.

   B. Identify which joints each crosses by indicating on the table below the position that would lengthen the muscle over each joint it crosses.

Lengthened Position at Each Joint the Muscle Crosses

Muscle	Elbow	Wrist	CMC	MP	PIP	DIP	IP

LAB ACTIVITIES
HAND

1. For each of the motions available at the carpometacarpal joint of the thumb,

   A. Place your open left hand in the correct orientation to represent the plane of a motion.

   B. Place your right index finger to indicate the axis of that plane of motion.

2. For each of the motions available at the joints listed below, estimate the degrees of motion available by checking the box that most closely describes the motion. (Do not use a goniometer.)

Carpometacarpal Joint of the Thumb

Motion	*0–45*	*46–90*	*91–135*	*136–180*
FLEXION				
EXTENSION				
ABDUCTION				
ADDUCTION				
OPPOSITION				

Metacarpophalangeal Joints of the Fingers 2-5

Motion	*0–45*	*46–90*	*91–135*	*136–180*
FLEXION				
HYPEREXTENSION				
ABDUCTION				
ADDUCTION				

Proximal Interphalangeal Joints

Motion	*0–45*	*46–90*	*91–135*	*136–180*
FLEXION				
HYPEREXTENSION				

Distal Interphalangeal Joints

Motion	*0–45*	*46–90*	*91–135*	*136–180*
FLEXION				
HYPEREXTENSION				

3. On the skeleton, anatomical models, and at least one partner, locate, palpate, and observe the structures described below. The reference position is the anatomical position. Having pictures for reference is helpful when trying to find the structures. Not all structures can be palpated on your partner.

Thumb

First metacarpal: Palpate by grasping the thumb just above the carpometacarpal joint.

Proximal phalange: Articulates with the first metacarpal bone and the distal phalange.

Distal phalange: Articulates with the proximal phalange of the thumb. The thumb has only two phalanges.

Carpometacarpal joint: Consists of the trapezium articulating with the base of the first metacarpal. Palpate the carpometacarpal joint on the palmar radial side of the hand at the wrist.

Metacarpophalangeal joint: Articulation of the first metacarpal with the proximal phalange. Commonly called "knuckles," they are the articulations between the metacarpals and the first phalanges.

Interphalangeal joint: Articulation of the proximal and distal phalanges.

Fingers: Second–Fifth digits

Metacarpals: The long bones of the hand that lie between the wrist and the fingers. The bases of the metacarpals articulate with the distal row of carpal bones. The heads of the metacarpals articulate with the proximal phalanges of the fingers.

Phalanges: The bones of the fingers. They are named by their location in relation to one another: Proximal, middle, and distal.

Carpometacarpal joints: The articulations of the proximal row of carpal bones with the metacarpal bones of the fingers. These joints are palpated more easily on the dorsum of the hand although they are covered by tendons on both the palmar and dorsal surfaces.

Metacarpophalangeal joints: Also called "knuckles," they are the articulations between the metacarpals and first phalanges. To palpate, make a fist and palpate the distal ends of the metacarpal bones on the dorsum of the hand. With your palpating fingers on the medial and lateral sides of the metacarpal, slide them just a short space distally. As you open your hand, feel the proximal phalange and the joint space.

Proximal interphalangeal joints: The articulation of the proximal and middle phalanges.

Distal interphalangeal joints: The articulation of the middle and distal phalanges.

4. On the skeleton, anatomical models, and at least one partner, locate the muscles listed below.

   A. Locate the origin and insertion of the muscle on the skeleton.

   B. Stretch a large rubber band taut by placing one end at the origin and the other end at the insertion of the muscle on the skeleton.

   C. Perform the motion that the muscle does and observe how the rubber band becomes less taut and shorter, similar to the muscle shortening as it contracts.

   D. Perform the opposite motion and observe how the rubber band becomes more taut and lengthened, similar to the muscle lengthening as it is stretched.

   E. After locating the muscle on the skeleton, locate the muscle on your partner. Not all origins, insertions, and muscle bellies can be palpated.

   F. When possible, palpate the origin, insertion, and muscle belly of each muscle by:

      1) Placing your fingers on the origin and insertion and asking your partner to contract the muscle.

      2) Moving your fingers from the origin to the insertion over the contracting muscle.

      3) Asking your partner to relax the muscle and again moving your fingers from the origin to the insertion over the muscle.

   All of these muscles can be examined with the individual in the sitting position.

   ### EXTRINSIC MUSCLES

   Flexor digitorum superficialis: Located deep to the wrist flexors and palmaris longus.

Position:	Sitting with the forearm supinated and the wrist in neutral.
Origin:	Common flexor tendon on the medial epicondyle of the humerus, coranoid process, and radius.
Insertion:	Sides of the middle phalanx of the four fingers.
Action:	Flex the MCP and PIP joints.
Palpate:	At the wrist lateral and deep to the palmaris longus.

   Flexor digitorum profundus: Located deep to the flexor digitorum superficialis.

Position:	Sitting with the forearm supinated and the wrist in neutral.
Origin:	Upper three-fourths of the ulna.
Insertion:	Distal phalanx of the four fingers.
Action:	Flex the DIP joint.
Palpate:	Difficult to palpate because it lies deep to other tendons on the anterior surface of the forearm.

   Extensor digitorum: Located superficially on the posterior forearm and hand.

Position:	Sitting with the forearm pronated and the wrist in neutral.
Origin:	Lateral epicondyle of the humerus.
Insertion:	Base of the distal phalanx second–fifth fingers.
Action:	Extend the MCP joints of the fingers.
Palpate:	Tendons on the dorsum of the hand.

Extensor digiti minimi: Located deep to the extensor digitorum and extensor carpi ulnaris muscles at the origin and superficial at the wrist.

Position:	Sitting with the forearm pronated and the wrist in neutral.
Origin:	Lateral epicondyle of the humerus.
Insertion:	Base of the distal phalanx of the fifth finger.
Action:	Extend the MCP joints of the fifth finger.
Palpate:	On the dorsum of the hand over the fifth finger lateral to the extensor digitorum.

Extensor indicis: Located deep on the posterior surface of the forearm.

Position:	Sitting with the forearm pronated and the wrist in neutral.
Origin:	Posterior surface of the distal ulna.
Insertion:	The extensor hood at the base of the distal phalange.
Action:	Extend the second MP joint.
Palpate:	The tendon on the dorsum of the hand over the second finger medial to the tendon of the extensor digitorum.

Flexor pollicis longus: Located deep on the anterior surface of the forearm.

Position:	Sitting with the forearm supinated and the wrist in neutral.
Origin:	Anterior surface of the radius.
Insertion:	Distal phalange of the thumb.
Action:	Flex the IP joint of the thumb.
Palpate:	The tendon on the palmar surface of the proximal phalange.

Abductor pollicis longus: Located deep on the posterior forearm.

Position:	Sitting with the forearm supinated and the wrist in neutral.
Origin:	Posterior surface of the radius, interosseous membrane, and posterior lateral surface of the middle portion of the ulna.
Insertion:	Radial side of the base of the first metacarpal.
Action:	Abduct the thumb.
Palpate:	At the insertion. This tendon lies next to the extensor pollicis brevis tendon to make up the lateral border of the anatomical snuffbox.

Extensor pollicis longus: Located deep on the posterior forearm.

Position:	Sitting with the forearm in midposition and the wrist in neutral.
Origin:	Posterior lateral side of the ulna and the interosseous membrane.
Insertion:	Base of the distal phalange of the thumb.
Action:	Extend the MCP and IP joints of the thumb.
Palpate:	The tendon on the dorsum of the proximal phalange. The extensor pollicis longus tendon is the tendon on the medial side (toward the second finger) of the anatomical snuffbox.

Extensor pollicis brevis: Located deep on the posterior distal forearm.

Position:	Sitting with the forearm in midposition and the wrist in neutral.
Origin:	Posterior distal surface of the radius.
Insertion:	Base of the proximal phalange of the thumb.
Action:	Extend the MP joint.
Palpate:	The tendon at the insertion. This tendon makes up the radial (thumb) side of the anatomical snuffbox.

Anatomical snuffbox: Located on the posterior radial side at the base of the thumb.

Action:	Extend the thumb.
Palpate:	The abductor pollicis longus and extensor pollicis brevis tendons on the radial side and the extensor pollicis longus tendon on the ulnar side.

INTRINSIC MUSCLES

Flexor pollicis brevis: Located superficially in the thenar group.

Position:	Sitting with the forearm supinated and the wrist in neutral.
Origin:	Trapezium, trapezoid, capitate, and flexor retinaculum.
Insertion:	Base of the proximal phalange of the thumb.
Action:	With the IP joint extended, flex the MP joint.
Palpate:	The muscle in the middle of the thenar eminence proximal to the metacarpophalangeal joint.

Abductor pollicis brevis: Located superficially in the thenar group.

Position:	Sitting with the forearm supinated and the wrist in neutral.
Origin:	Scaphoid, trapezium, and the flexor retinaculum.
Insertion:	Radial side of the base of the proximal phalanx.
Action:	Abduct the thumb.
Palpate:	The muscle belly in the thenar eminence on the lateral aspect of the first metacarpal.

Opponens pollicis: Located deep in the palm.

Position:	Sitting with the forearm supinated and the wrist in neutral.
Origin:	Trapezium and flexor retinaculum.
Insertion:	First metacarpal.
Action:	Oppose the thumb and little finger by touching the pad of the thumb to the pad of the little finger.
Palpate:	On the radial side of the first metacarpal lateral to the abductor pollicis brevis.

Adductor pollicis: Located deep on the thenar side.

Position:	Sitting with the forearm pronated and the wrist in neutral.
Origin:	Capitate, base of the second metacarpal, and palmar surface of the third metacarpal.
Insertion:	Base of the proximal phalange of the thumb.
Action:	Adduct the thumb.
Palpate:	In the web space between the first and second metacarpals.

Flexor digiti minimi: Located in the hypothenar eminence.

Position: Sitting with the forearm supinated and the wrist in neutral.
Origin: Hamate and flexor retinaculum.
Insertion: Base of the proximal phalange of the fifth finger.
Action: Flex the MCP joint.
Palpate: The muscle belly in the hypothenar eminence on the anterior surface over the distal end of the fifth metacarpal.

Abductor digiti minimi: Located superficially on the ulnar border of the hypothenar eminence.

Position: Sitting with the forearm pronated and the wrist in neutral.
Origin: Pisiform and tendon of the flexor carpi ulnaris.
Insertion: Medial side of the base of the proximal phalange of the fifth finger.
Action: Abduct the fifth finger.
Palpate: The muscle on the medial (ulnar) aspect of the fifth metacarpal.

Opponens digiti minimi: Located deep to the other hypothenar muscles.

Position: Sitting with the forearm supinated and the wrist in neutral.
Origin: Hamate and flexor retinaculum.
Insertion: Medial side of the fifth metacarpal.
Action: Oppose the fifth finger by touching the pad of the fifth finger to the pad of the thumb.
Palpate: In the hypothenar eminence on the anterior surface over the proximal end of the fifth metacarpal.

Dorsal interossei: Located deep on the dorsum of the hand.

Position: Sitting with the forearm pronated and the wrist in neutral.

Muscle	Origin	Insertion	Action: Abduct
1st	1st and 2nd metacarpals	Lateral side of proximal phalanx of index finger	Index finger
2nd	2nd and 3rd metacarpals	Lateral side of proximal phalanx of middle finger	Middle finger laterally
3rd	3rd and 4th metacarpals	Medial side of proximal phalanx of middle finger	Middle finger medially
4th	4th and 5th metacarpals	Medial side of proximal phalanx of ring finger	Ring finger

Palpation of the second, third, and fourth dorsal interossei is not possible. The first dorsal interossei can be palpated at the base of the proximal phalange.

Palmar interossei: Located deep in the palm.

Position: Sitting with the forearm supinated and the wrist in neutral.

Muscle	Origin	Insertion	Action: Adduct
1st	1st metacarpal	Medial side of thumb	Thumb
2nd	2nd metacarpal	Medial side of index finger	Index finger
3rd	4th metacarpal	Lateral side of ring finger	Ring finger
4th	5th metacarpal	Lateral side of little finger	Little finger

Palpation: Is not possible.

Lumbricales: Located deep on the lateral side.

Position: Sitting with the forearm pronated and the wrist in neutral.
Origin: Tendons of the flexor digitorum profundus muscle.
Insertion: Radial side of the corresponding digit's extensor hood.
Action: Flex the MP joints with extension of the IP joints.
Palpation: Is not possible.

5. Referring to question 9 in the Worksheets, assume the positions that lengthen the extrinsic hand muscles simultaneously over the joints they cross.

6. Observe the transverse and longitudinal palmar arches. The transverse arch is observed as the medial-lateral arch, or curve of the palm of the hand. The longitudinal arch is the proximal-distal arch, or curve of the palm of the hand. These arches are formed by the shape of the bones of the hand and the relative lengths of the palmar and dorsal ligaments and fascia.

7. PALMAR CREASES (Outline with different colored pens.)

   Radial longitudinal crease: Outlines the thenar eminence.

   Midpalmar crease: Outlines the hypothenar eminence.

   Proximal transverse crease: Is located in the midpalmar area.

   Distal transverse crease: Is located near the heads of the metacarpals.

   A. Observe the creases on the palmar surface of the hand and on the palmar and dorsal surfaces of the fingers.

   B. Describe the general locations and directions of the creases: _____

   _____

   _____

   _____

   C. Describe what happens to the creases as the fingers are flexed and extended. _____

   _____

   _____

   _____

8. A. Perform wrist flexion and extension with the MCP and IP joints flexed.

   B. Repeat with the MCP and IP joints extended.

   C. Observe the range of wrist motion available under each condition.

   D. Describe how the positions of the MP and IP joints affect the range of wrist motion. _____

   _____

   _____

   _____

   E. Explain your observations. _____

   _____

9. Perform each of the following types of grasp. Describe one functional task performed with each type of grasp.

   A. **Cylindrical grasp:** Fingers are adducted and flexed around the object with the thumb adducted.

   Example: _____

   B. **Spherical grasp:** Fingers flexed and abducted around the object with the thumb opposed.

   Example: _____

   C. **Hook grasp:** Fingers are flexed at the interphalangeal joints only and the thumb does not participate.

   Example: _____

   D. **Lateral prehension:** Pad of thumb is flexed against the lateral aspect of the index finger.

   Example: _____

   E. **Tip-to-tip prehension:** Tip of thumb is touched to tip of finger, usually the index finger.

   Example: _____

   F. **Pad-to-pad prehension:** Pad of thumb is touched to pad of finger.

   Example: _____

10. Describe the conditions that permit the extensor muscles of the wrist to produce grasp. _____

    _____

    _____

    _____

11. Hold a piece of paper between your index and middle fingers, or any other two adjacent fingers, while your classmate tries to pull the paper out from in between your fingers.

    A. Could the paper be removed easily? _____

    B. Which muscles were at work and what were their actions? _____

    _____

    C. Damage to which nerve would weaken these muscles?_____

POST-LAB QUESTIONS
HAND

After you have completed the Worksheets and Lab Activities, answer the following questions without using your books or notes. When finished, check your answers.

1. Identify the following muscles by their location to each other.
    A. What is the most superficial muscle on the anterior surface of the wrist located in the midline at the wrist?_____

    B. What muscle or tendon lies directly underneath the muscle identified in A?_____

    _____

    C. What muscle or tendon lies directly underneath the muscle identified in B?_____

    _____

2. What is the difference between an extrinsic muscle and an intrinsic muscle? _____

    _____

    _____

3. Are thenar and hypothenar muscles intrinsic or extrinsic muscles?_____

4. A. List the muscles that make up the anatomical snuffbox. _____

    _____

    B. Are these muscles intrinsic or extrinsic muscles? _____

5. Which muscle attaches to the tendons of the flexor digitorum profundus and extensor digitorum muscles? _____

6. A. A "thenar" muscle is going to have an action on what structure? _____

    B. The thenar eminence consists of which muscles?_____

    _____

    C. Which nerve innervates the muscles of the thenar eminence?_____

    D. Which thumb motions would be affected by damage to this nerve?_____

    _____

7. If one were to generalize about the innervation of the muscles of the hand by their location, the muscles on the:
    A. Posterior surface are innervated by the _____.
    B. Anterior medial surface are innervated by the _____.
    C. Anterior lateral surface are innervated by the _____.

8. An individual with a nerve injury that eliminates thumb opposition has injured which nerve?

   _____

9. A. Which muscles have the combined action of MP flexion and IP extension?_____

   _____

   B. Give one example of using this action in a functional activity. _____

   _____

10. What is the reference point for MP abduction and adduction? _____

11. A. Compared to the fingers, what bone is the thumb missing? _____

    B. What is the effect of this missing bone on the number of joints? _____

    _____

    C. What motion does the thumb have that fingers two to four do not have? _____

12. All joints of the thumb and fingers are what type of joints? _____

13. A. Which extrinsic muscles of the hand are involved in extension of the fingers?_____

    _____

    B. Which extrinsic muscles of the hand are involved in flexion of the fingers? _____

    _____

14. Which muscle abducts the index finger?_____

9

HIP JOINT

Student's Name _____   Date Due _____

WORKSHEETS

Complete the following questions prior to lab class.

1. On the drawings,

   A. Label the bones and landmarks.

   ILIUM

   Iliac crest
   Anterior superior iliac spine
   Anterior inferior iliac spine
   Posterior superior iliac spine
   Posterior inferior iliac spine

   ISCHIUM

   Ramus
   Ischial tuberosity
   Body

   PUBIS

   Body
   Superior ramus
   Inferior ramus
   Pubic tubercle

   ILIUM, ISCHIUM, AND/OR PUBIS

   Acetabulum
   Obturator foramen
   Greater sciatic notch

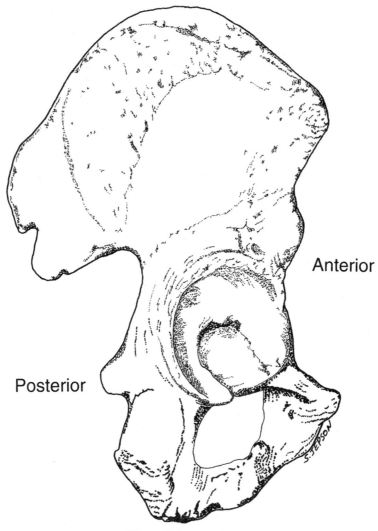

Anterior

Posterior

Figure 9.1 *Lateral view.*

ILIUM, ISCHIUM, AND/OR PUBIS

Acetabulum
Obturator foramen
Iliac fossa
Symphysis pubis

SACRUM
COCCYX

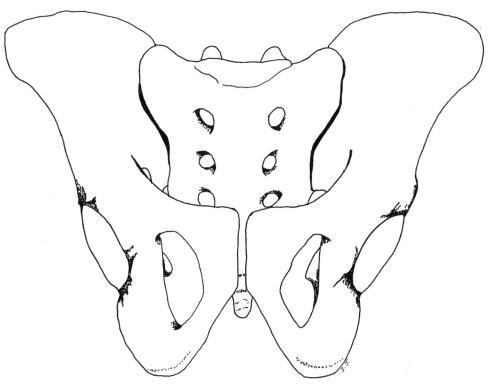

Figure 9.2 *Anterior view.*

FEMUR

Head   Neck
Greater trochanter   Lesser trochanter
Shaft   Medial condyle
Lateral condyle   Lateral epicondyle
Medial epicondyle   Adductor tubercle
Linea aspera   Patellar surface
Attachment of ligamentum teres

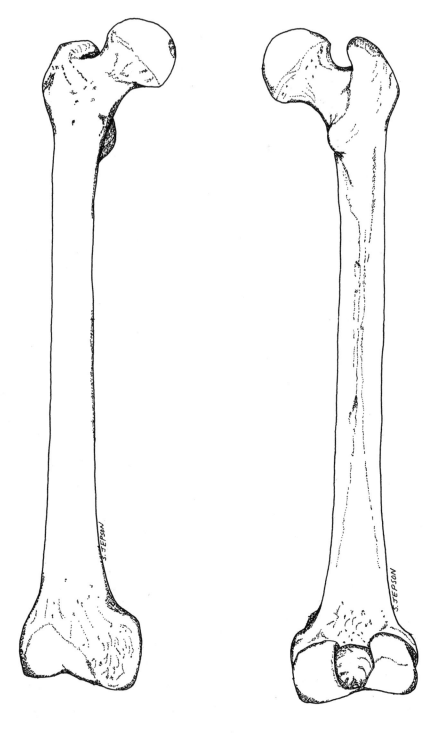

Anterior   Posterior

Figure 9.3 *Anterior and posterior femur.*

TIBIA

Tuberosity

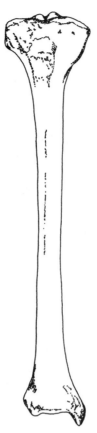

Figure 9.4 *Tibia, anterior view.*

B. Draw in the soft tissue structures and label the joints.

Joint capsule
Inguinal ligament

Pubofemoral ligament
Iliofemoral ligament

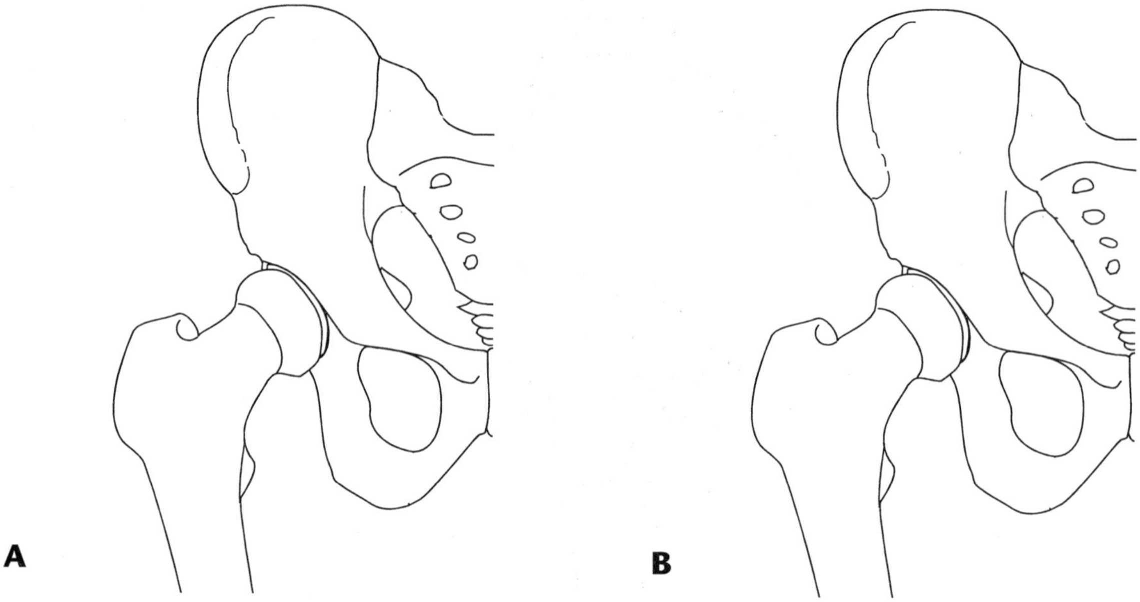

A

B

Figure 9.5 *(A) and (B) Anterior view.*

Ischiofemoral ligament

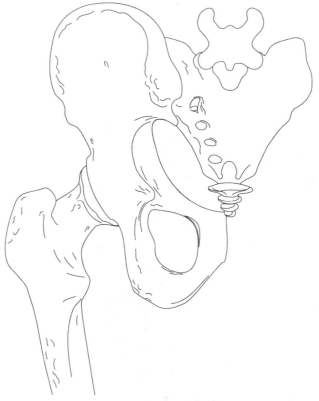

Figure 9.6 *Posterior view.*

Hip joint
Iliotibial band/tract
Knee joint

Femur
Tibia
Fibula

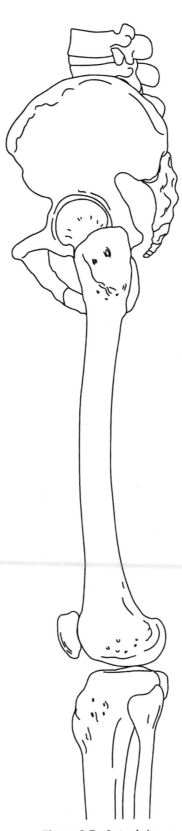

Figure 9.7 *Lateral view.*

2. On the drawings,

A. Label the origin and insertion of the muscles indicated.
   Color the origin in red and the insertion in blue.

B. Join the origin and insertion to show the muscle belly.

Iliopsoas

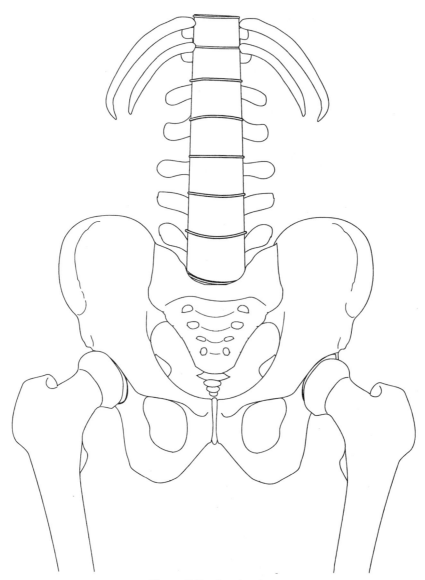

Figure 9.8 *Anterior view.*

Rectus femoris

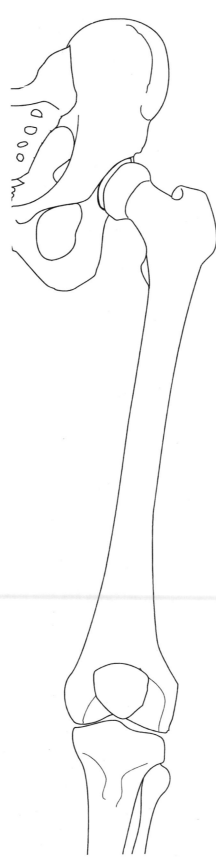

Figure 9.9 _Anterior view._

Sartorius

Pectineus

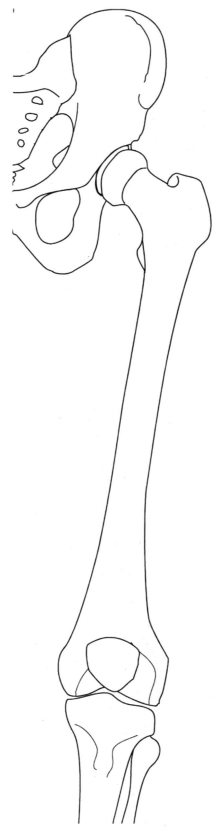

Figure 9.10 *Anterior view.*

Gracilis

Adductor longus

Adductor brevis

Adductor magnus

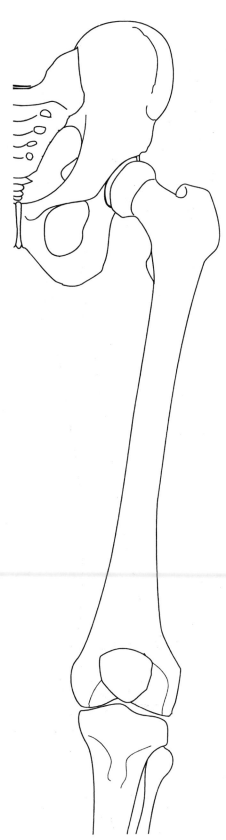

Figure 9.11 *Anterior view.*

Gluteus maximus

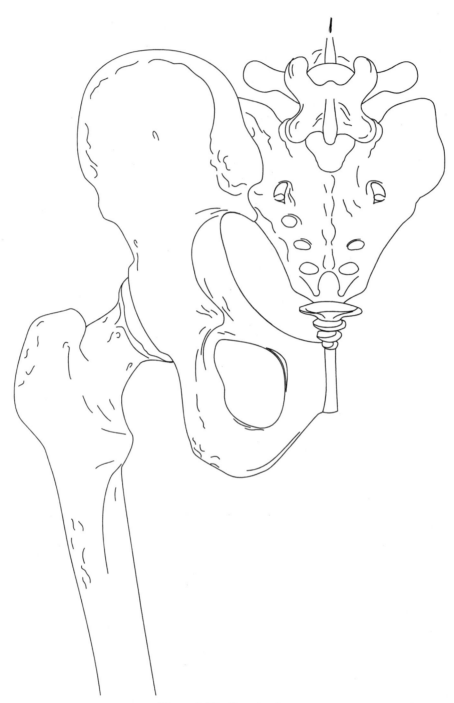

Figure 9.12 *Posterior view.*

Semimembranosus

Semitendinosus

Biceps femoris

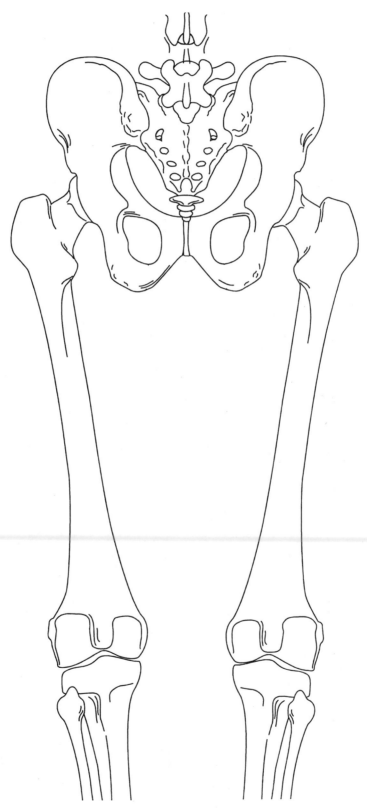

Figure 9.13 *Posterior view.*

Gluteus medius

Gluteus minimus

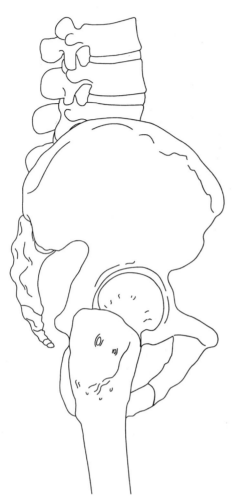

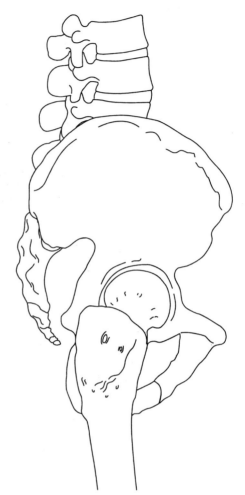

Figure 9.14 *Lateral view.*

Figure 9.15 *Lateral view.*

Tensor fascia latea

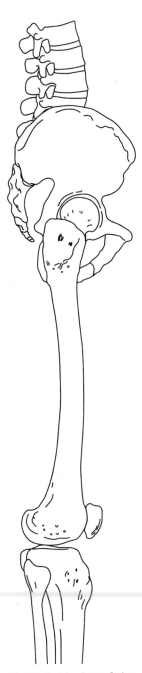

Figure 9.16 *Lateral view.*

3. For the hip joint, identify the following.

Shape	Number of Axes

4. Name the structure of the hip joint that is concave. _____

   Name the structure of the hip joint that is convex. _____

5. Match each ligament and structure listed to its function. Use each answer only once.

   _____ Joint capsule

   _____ Iliofemoral ligament

   _____ Pubofemoral ligament

   _____ Ischiofemoral ligament

   _____ Ligamentum teres

   _____ Acetabular labrum

   _____ Inguinal ligament

   _____ Iliotibial band

   A. Reinforce hip joint capsule anteriorly
   B. Contains blood vessels to the femoral head
   C. Encases head and neck of femur
   D. Limits abduction of hip joint
   E. Is insertion for gluteus maximus and tensor fascia latae muscle
   F. Assists to hold head in acetabulum
   G. Reinforce hip joint capsule posteriorly
   H. Is landmark denoting separation of trunk from the lower extremity

6. For the hip joint, indicate which *motions* are available, in which *plane* the motion occurs, and the *axis* of each motion.

Motion	Plane	Axis

7. For each hip motion listed, *check* the muscle(s) that are major contributors to that action.

Motion	Iliopsoas	Rectus femoris	Sartorius	Pectineus	Adductor magnus	Adductor longus	Adductor brevis	Gracilis
FLEXION								
EXTENSION								
HYPEREXTENSION								
ABDUCTION								
ADDUCTION								
MEDIAL ROTATION								
LATERAL ROTATION								

Motion	Gluteus maximus	Gluteus medius	Gluteus minimus	Semi-membranous	Semi-tendinous	Biceps femoris	Tensor fascia latae	Deep rotator group
FLEXION								
EXTENSION								
HYPEREXTENSION								
ABDUCTION								
ADDUCTION								
MEDIAL ROTATION								
LATERAL ROTATION								

8. A. List the multijoint muscles of the hip

   B. Identify the action of each muscle at each joint it crosses.

Muscle	Trunk	Hip	Knee

9. Describe the positions that make the:

   A. Hamstrings, actively insufficient:_____

   B. Hamstrings, passively insufficient: _____

   C. Rectus femoris, actively insufficient:_____

   D. Rectus femoris, passively insufficient:_____

LAB ACTIVITIES
HIP JOINT

1. For each of the motions available at the hip joint, estimate the degrees of motion available by checking the box which most closely describes that motion. (Do not use a goniometer.)

Motion	*0–45*	*46–90*	*91–135*	*136–180*
FLEXION				
HYPEREXTENSION				
ABDUCTION				
ADDUCTION				
MEDIAL ROTATION				
LATERAL ROTATION				

2. On the skeleton, anatomical models, and at least one partner, locate, palpate, and observe the structures described below. The reference position is the anatomical position. Having pictures for reference is helpful when trying to find the structures. Not all structures can be palpated.

Ilium

Iliac fossa: Located on the internal surface of the ilium. It is the large concave portion of the internal surface of the ilium. It cannot be palpated.

Iliac crest: The superior portion of the ilium between the posterior superior iliac spine to the anterior superior iliac spine. It is the bony structure just below your waist. Palpate the entire crest by moving from the anterior superior iliac spine to the posterior superior iliac spine. The iliac crests appear to be located more superiorly on men than women.

Anterior superior iliac spine (ASIS): This protuberance is located on the anterior of the ilium marking the anterior border of the iliac crest. It is the attachment for the tensor fascia latea and sartorius muscles and the inguinal ligament. To palpate, place your hand on the iliac crest and move anteriorly to the anteriormost point, which is the ASIS.

Anterior inferior iliac spine (AIIS): Located on the anterior of the ilium inferior to the ASIS. It is the attachment for the rectus femoris muscle. The AIIS is inferior to the ASIS and deep to several muscles making palpation difficult.

Posterior superior iliac spine (PSIS): The superior protuberance on the posterior of the ilium marking the posterior border of the iliac crest. To palpate, place your hands on the iliac crest and move posteriorly and medially. The first protuberance felt is the PSIS. A "dimple" is usually observable over the PSIS.

Posterior inferior iliac spine (PIIS): The inferior protuberance on the posterior of the ilium. It is inferior to the PSIS.

Ischium:

Body: Located posteriorly and inferiorly on the ischium comprising about two-fifths of the acetabulum. It cannot be palpated.

Ramus: Extends anteriorly from the body to connect with the inferior ramus of the pubis. The adductor magnus, obturator externus, and obturator internus attach on the ischial ramus. Palpation is not usually possible.

Ischial tuberosity: Located on the inferior body of the ischium. It is the blunt bony projection upon which one sits. Several muscles attach to the ischial tuberosity including the hamstrings and adductor magnus. It can often be palpated by having your partner sit on your fingers. Another method is to palpate the ischium while your partner flexes the trunk on the thigh in the standing position. This method is used to check the fit of an above-knee prosthesis.

Pubis

Body: Located anteriorly. The body forms one-fifth of the acetabulum and is the attachment for the obturator internus (deep rotator) muscle. It is adjacent to the pubic symphysis. Palpation is possible but not usually performed.

Superior ramus: Located superiorly between the acetabulum and the body. It provides attachment for the pectineus muscle. Palpation is not usually possible.

Inferior ramus: Located posterior, inferior, and lateral to the body. The gracilis and adductors magnus and brevis attach to it. Palpation is not usually possible.

Symphysis pubis: Located at the anterior midline of the body. It is the cartilaginous joint that joins the right and left pubic bones. Palpation is not usually possible.

Pubic tubercle: The anterior protuberance on the superior ramus close to the pubic symphysis. It is the attachment for the inguinal ligament and is not easily palpated.

Ilium, Ischium, and Pubis Combined

Acetabulum: Located on the lateral aspect of the pelvis. It is a deep cavity forming the pelvic part of the hip joint. It cannot be palpated.

Obturator foramen: Located inferior to the acetabulum, it is a large opening formed by the bodies and rami of the ischium and pubis, through which blood vessels and nerves pass. It cannot be palpated.

Greater sciatic notch: Located posteriorly, it is a large notch just below the PIIS through which passes the sciatic nerve and piriformis muscle. It is not easily palpated.

Femur

Head: Located medially on the proximal end of the femur, it is the smooth rounded portion of the femur that articulates with the acetabulum. It cannot be palpated.

Neck: Located near the proximal end, it is the narrow portion lateral to the head and between the head and the trochanters. It cannot be palpated.

Greater trochanter: The large protuberance on the proximal lateral aspect of the femur. The gluteus medius and minimus and most deep rotator muscles attach to it. It is easily palpated on the proximal lateral aspect of the femur. Medial and lateral rotation of the hip will cause it to rotate anteriorly and posteriorly, allowing it to be palpated as it rolls under your fingers.

Lesser trochanter: The smaller protuberance located on the proximal medial aspect of the femur. It is the attachment of the iliopsoas muscle making palpation difficult.

Shaft: The long cylindrical portion also known as the body. It is almost completely covered by muscle and cannot be palpated.

Medial condyle: The enlargement on the distal medial side of the femur where it is palpated just proximal to the knee joint.

Lateral condyle: The enlargement on the distal lateral side of the femur where it can be palpated just proximal to the knee joint.

Lateral epicondyle: The projection on the lateral side proximal to the lateral condyle. It is not readily distinguishable with palpation.

Medial epicondyle: The projection proximal to the medial condyle. It is not readily distinguishable with palpation.

Adductor tubercle: The small projection proximal to the medial epicondyle providing attachment for the adductor magnus muscle. Because of the muscles in the area, the adductor tubercle is not easily palpated.

Linea aspera: Located on the posterior surface is a long prominent longitudinal ridge or crest. Because of the muscles overlying the area, it cannot be palpated.

Patellar surface: An area located on the distal anterior surface between the condyles that articulates with the patella. When the knee is fully flexed and the patella has moved distally, part of the patellar surface can be palpated.

Tibia (will be covered in detail in next chapter)

Tibial tuberosity: A large projection located in the midline on the proximal anterior aspect of the tibia. The quadriceps muscle tendon inserts on the tibial tuberosity via the patellar tendon. Often the tibial tuberosity is visually evident. To palpate, place your fingers on the midline of the tibia distal to the knee joint. Asking your partner to extend his or her knee will make it easier to locate because knee extension will cause the tendon to become taut and thus more prominent.

Other Structures

Joint capsule: A strong thick fibrous cylindrical sleeve that encloses the joint and most of the femoral neck. Because it is a deep structure, it cannot be palpated. It is reinforced by three ligaments.

Iliofemoral ligament: Crosses the joint anteriorly from the AIIS to the intertrochanteric line of the femur—a line between the greater and lesser trochanters. Because the ligament splits before inserting on the femur, it resembles the letter "Y" and is often referred to as the "Y" ligament. Another name is the "ligament of Bigelow." Being a deep structure, it cannot be palpated.

Pubofemoral ligament: Crosses the hip joint on the medial inferior side. It passes posteriorly and inferiorly from the medial aspect of the acetabular rim and superior ramus of the pubis to the neck of the femur. Being a deep structure, it cannot be palpated.

Ischiofemoral ligament: Crosses the hip joint on the posterior side where it attaches on the ischial portion of the acetabulum. It passes in a lateral and superior direction to insert on the femoral neck. Being a deep structure, it cannot be palpated.

Ligamentum teres: The small intracapsular ligament attaches to the acetabulum and the fovea of the femoral head. The function is not entirely clear. It is within the hip joint (intercapsular) and cannot be palpated.

Acetabular labrum: Located around the rim of the acetabulum, it serves to increase the depth of the acetabulum and surround the head of the femur, holding the head in the acetabulum. Being a deep structure, it cannot be palpated.

Inguinal ligament: Located on the anterior surface, it serves as the boundary between the trunk and lower extremity. It attaches to the ASIS and the pubic tubercle. The femoral artery and vein pass under the inguinal ligament. Palpate the femoral pulse and move your fingers proximally to the inguinal ligament.

Iliotibial band: Located on the lateral aspect of the thigh attaching to the anterior portion of the iliac crest and the proximal anterolateral tibia. Fibers of the gluteus maximus and tensor fascia latae muscles insert into the iliotibial band. Placing the hip in extension and adduction causes the iliotibial band to become taut and easier to palpate.

3. Locate the muscles listed below on the skeleton and on at least one partner.

   A. Locate the origin and insertion of the muscle on the skeleton.

   B. Stretch a large rubber band taut by placing one end at the origin and the other end at the insertion of the muscle on the skeleton.

   C. Perform the motion that muscle does and observe how the rubber band becomes less taut and shorter, similar to the muscle shortening as it contracts.

   D. Perform the opposite motion and observe how the rubber band becomes more taut and longer, similar to the muscle lengthening as it is stretched.

   E. After locating the muscle on the skeleton, locate the muscle on your partner. The position described for locating the muscle on your partner is the manual muscle test position for a fair or better grade of muscle strength. Not all origins, insertions, and muscle bellies can be palpated on your partner.

   F. When possible, palpate the origin, insertion, and muscle belly of each muscle by:

      1) Placing your fingers on the origin and insertion and asking your partner to contract the muscle.

      2) Moving your fingers from the origin to the insertion over the contracting muscle.

      3) Asking your partner to relax the muscle and again moving your fingers from the origin to the insertion over the muscle.

SITTING POSITION

Iliopsoas: Located deep on the anterior aspect of the hip joint.

Position:	Sitting on the side of the treatment table.
Origin:	Anterior surface of the iliac fossa, the anterior and lateral surfaces of the vertebral bodies and the transverse processes of T12 to L5.
Insertion:	Lesser trochanter of the femur.
Action:	Flex the hip by lifting the thigh off the supporting surface without rotation.
Palpate:	At the midline in the "bend" of the hip, distal to the inguinal ligament.

Rectus femoris: Located superficially on the anterior of the thigh. This muscle is part of the quadriceps muscle.

Position:	Sitting on the side of the treatment table.
Origin:	Anterior inferior iliac spine.
Insertion:	Tibial tuberosity via the patellar tendon.
Action:	Flex the hip by lifting the thigh off the supporting surface without rotation.
Palpate:	Lateral to the iliopsas. As part of the quadriceps, this muscle flexes the hip.

Sartorius: Located superficially anterior to the hip joint and medially on the thigh.

Position:	Sitting on the side of the treatment table.
Origin:	Anterior superior iliac spine.
Insertion:	Proximal medial aspect of the tibia.
Action:	Flex, abduct, and laterally rotate the hip.
Palpate:	Near the origin and as it crosses diagonally to the medial side of the thigh.

Deep rotator muscles: Located deep. These muscles will be treated as a group. The muscles included are:

Obturator externus	Obturator internus
Quadratus femoris	Piriformis
Gemellus superior	Gemellus inferior

Position: Sitting on the side of the treatment table.
Origins: Posterior sacrum, ischium, and pubis.
Insertions: Greater trochanter area.
Action: Externally rotate the hip by moving the foot in and up.
Palpate: These deep muscles cannot be palpated.

SIDE LYING POSITION ON SAME SIDE AS MUSCLE BEING EXAMINED

Pectineus: Located deep and inferior to the hip joint.

Position: Side lying on the side being examined.
Origin: Superior ramus of the pubis.
Insertion: Pectineal line of the femur.
Action: Adduct the hip by lifting the leg off the table.
Palpate: On the proximal medial aspect of the thigh.

Gracilis: Located superficially on the medial aspect of the thigh.

Position: Side lying on the side to be examined.
Origin: Pubis.
Insertion: Anterior medial surface of the proximal tibia below the tibial plateau.
Action: Adduct the hip lifting the leg off the table.
Palpate: On the medial aspect of the thigh. Because the adductors are relatively close together and all perform the same action, distinguishing between the muscles can be difficult.

Adductor magnus: Located on the medial aspect of the thigh deep to the adductor longus and brevis, and gracilis.

Position: Side lying on the side to be examined.
Origin: Ischial tuberosity and pubis.
Insertion: Linea aspera and adductor tubercle of the medial condyle of the femur.
Action: Adduct the hip by lifting the leg off the table.
Palpate: On the distal medial aspect of the thigh.

Adductor longus: Located superficially on the medial aspect of the thigh.

Position: Side lying on the side to be examined.
Origin: Anterior crest of the pubis.
Insertion: Middle one-third of the linea aspera of the femur.
Action: Adduct the hip by lifting the leg off the table.
Palpate: On the proximal anterior medial aspect of the groin. This tendon is usually prominent and important to check as part of determining the correct fit of the quadrilateral socket of the above-knee prosthesis.

Adductor brevis: Located deep to the adductor longus on the medial aspect of the thigh.

Position: Side lying on the side to be examined.
Origin: Body and inferior surface of the pubis.
Insertion: Pectineal line and proximal linea aspera of the femur.
Action: Adduct the hip by lifting the leg off the table.
Palpate: On the proximal medial aspect of the thigh. It is difficult to distinguish between the adductor muscles.

PRONE POSITION

Gluteus maximus: Located superficially on the posterior surface of the pelvis.

Position:	Prone hip and knee extended.
Origin:	Posterior surfaces of the sacrum, ilium, and coccyx.
Insertion:	Posterior femur distal to the greater trochanter and the iliotibial band.
Action:	With the knee flexed, extend the hip by lifting the leg off the table.
Palpate:	With firm pressure on the center of the buttocks.

Semitendinosus: Located superficially on the posterior medial aspect of the thigh.

Position:	Prone hip and knee extended.
Origin:	Ischial tuberosity.
Insertion:	Anteromedial surface of the proximal tibia.
Action:	Extend the hip by lifting the leg off the table.
Palpate:	This muscle has a long distal tendon and can be palpated superficial to the semimembranosus.

Semimembranosus: Located deep to the semitendinosus on the posterior medial aspect of the thigh.

Position:	Prone hip and knee extended.
Origin:	Ischial tuberosity.
Insertion:	Posterior surface of the medial condyle of the tibia.
Action:	Extend the hip by lifting the leg off the table.
Palpate:	Distinguishing between the semimembranosus and semitendinosus can be difficult. The semimembranosus has a broad insertion on the posterior medial surface of the tibia deep to, and on either side of, the semitendinosus just above the bend of the knee. It is at this location where the distinction between the two muscles is easiest.

Biceps femoris: Located superficially on the posterior lateral thigh.

Position:	Prone hip and knee extended.
Origin:	Long head: Ischial tuberosity. Short head: Lateral lip of the linea aspera of the femur.
Insertion:	Posterior proximal fibular head.
Action:	Extend the hip by lifting the leg off the table.
Palpate:	Its distal tendon can be palpated on the lateral side just above the bend of the knee.

SIDE LYING POSITION ON SIDE OPPOSITE MUSCLE BEING EXAMINED

Gluteus medius: Located partially superficial and partially deep to the gluteus maximus.

Position:	Side lying with the top leg being examined.
Origin:	Outer surface of the ilium.
Insertion:	Greater trochanter of the femur.
Action:	Abduct the hip, moving the leg toward the ceiling.
Palpate:	On the lateral aspect of the ilium proximal to its insertion. It may be difficult to distinguish it from the gluteus minimus.

Gluteus minimus: Located deep to the gluteus medius.

Position:	Side lying with the top leg being examined.
Origin:	Outer surface of the ilium and greater sciatic notch.

Insertion:	Greater trochanter of the femur.
Action:	Abduct the hip, moving the leg towards the ceiling.
Palpate:	On the lateral aspect of the ilium proximal to the insertion. It may be difficult to distinguish it from the gluteus medius.

Tensor fascia latae: Located superficially.

Position:	Side lying with the top leg being examined and in approximately 45 degrees of flexion.
Origin:	Anterior superior iliac spine and the iliac crest.
Insertion:	Lateral condyle of the tibia.
Action:	Flex and abduct the hip, moving the leg slightly forward and toward the ceiling.
Palpate:	On the proximal anterolateral aspect of the thigh distal to the ASIS.

4. Refer to Worksheet question 8, if necessary:

   A. Assume the positions that shorten the multijoint muscles simultaneously over all the joints they cross.

   B. Assume the positions that lengthen the multijoint muscles simultaneously over all the joints they cross.

5. Use a disarticulated skeleton or model of the hip joint and apply the rules of joint arthrokinematics and the concave-convex rule to perform the following exercise.

   A. Move the distal bone, the femur, on the proximal bone, the pelvis, in all planes of motion. This is an open kinetic chain activity.

   B. Observe the movement of the proximal end of the femur and then circle the motions that you observed.

   Spin   Roll   Glide   None

   C. Observe the direction of movement of the proximal end of the femur in relation to the movement of the distal end of femur as you move the femur in the acetabulum. Does the distal end of the femur move in the same direction or in the opposite direction as the proximal end of the femur? _____

6. Diagram the lever that describes *abduction of the right lower extremity* through its full range of motion when in the standing position.

   A. On the figure, label the Xs that represent the axis, muscle, and gravity, and identify the specific joint and muscle group.

   B. Make arrows out of the vertical lines to indicate the direction of the movement, the direction of the pull of the muscle, and the direction of the gravity.

   C. Identify the muscle and gravity as either *force* or *resistance*.

X	X	X	Direction of movement

7. A. Which joint motion is being analyzed? _____

   B. Identify the "axis" of the motion. _____

   C. Is the "force" causing the movement a muscle or gravity? _____

   D. Is the "resistance" to the movement a muscle or gravity? _____

   E. Which major muscle group is the agonist? _____

   F. Which major muscle group is the antagonist? _____

   G. Is the muscle acting to overcome gravity or slow down gravity? _____

   H. Is the agonist performing an isometric or isotonic contraction? _____

   I. If isotonic, is the agonist performing a concentric or an eccentric contraction? _____

   J. Is this an open or closed kinetic chain activity? _____

8. Diagram the lever that describes *adduction of the right lower extremity* from the fully abducted position to the anatomical position when in the standing position.

    A. On the figure, label the Xs that represent the axis, muscle, and gravity, and identify the specific joint and muscle group.

    B. Make arrows out of the vertical lines to indicate the direction of the movement, the direction of the pull of the muscle, and the direction of gravity.

    C. Identify the muscle and gravity as either *force* or *resistance*.

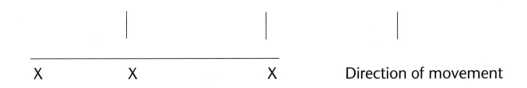

9. A. Which joint motion is being analyzed?_____

    B. Identify the "axis" of the motion. _____

    C. Is the "force" causing the movement a muscle or gravity?_____

    D. Is the "resistance" to the movement a muscle or gravity? _____

    E. Which major muscle group is the agonist?_____

    F. Which major muscle group is the antagonist?_____

    G. Is the muscle acting to overcome gravity or slow down gravity? _____

    H. Is the agonist performing an isometric or isotonic contraction?_____

    I. If isotonic, is the agonist performing a concentric or an eccentric contraction? _____

    J. Is this an open or closed kinetic chain activity? _____

10. Diagram the lever that describes the activity in the frontal plane of the *left hip* when, in the *standing position,* the *right lower extremity is abducted* through its full range of motion.

    A. On the figure, label the Xs that represent the axis, muscle, and gravity, and identify the specific joint and muscle group.

    B. Make arrows out of the vertical lines to indicate the direction of the movement, the direction of the pull of the muscle, and the direction of gravity.

    C. Identify the muscle and gravity as either *force* or *resistance*.

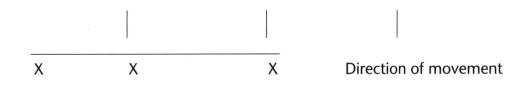

11. A. Which joint motion is being analyzed? _____

   B. Identify the "axis" of the motion. _____

   C. Which major muscle group is the agonist? _____

   D. Which major muscle group is the antagonist? _____

   E. Is the agonist performing an isotonic or an isometric contraction? _____

     If isotonic, is the agonist performing a concentric or an eccentric contraction? _____

   F. Is this an open or closed kinetic chain activity? _____

Student's Name _____ Date Due _____

POST-LAB QUESTIONS
HIP JOINT

After you have completed the Worksheets and Lab Activities, answer the following questions without using your books or notes. When finished, check your answers.

1. In the sitting position,

    A. List the combined joint actions required to put your right ankle on your left knee.

    _____

    B. Give the muscle that does the actions described in A. _____

    _____

2. Which hip muscle has an attachment on the spine? _____

3. List, in order, the hip muscles that have an attachment below the knee, starting at the anterior midline and proceding laterally around the knee. _____

    _____

4. Generally speaking, the following muscles share innervation from which peripheral nerve:

    Hamstrings: _____

    Hip flexors: _____

    Hip adductors: _____

5. When applying a hot-pack treatment to the buttock area, list the muscles in the order in which they will be heated if the heat penetrates from the most superficial muscle to the deepest.

    _____

    _____

6. The acetabulum is the _____ surface of the hip joint and the _____ _____ is the convex surface.

7. You are working with a patient with a hip problem. As you observe the patient you need to know the muscles that attach to the ischial tuberosity. List the muscles that attach to the ischial tuberosity. _____

    _____

8. Of the deep rotators of the hip, the piriformis is clinically significant because it can cause compression of a peripheral nerve. Which nerve is in a position to be compressed by the piriformis muscle? _____

9. Comparing the structures of hip and shoulder joints, give two reasons why the hip joint is a much more stable joint than the shoulder joint._____

_____

10. You are to position a patient side lying. What superficial bony landmark located on the proximal lateral aspect of the thigh may need to be padded to prevent development of a pressure sore?

_____

11. As you are observing a patient with anterior hip pain, you review the muscles in the area. List the muscles that share a common attachment on the anterior superior iliac spine. _____

_____

10

KNEE JOINT

Student's Name _____   Date Due _____

WORKSHEETS

Complete the following questions prior to lab class.

1. On the drawings,

    A. Label the joints, bones, and major landmarks.

TIBIA	Intercondylar eminence	Tibial tuberosity
	Medial condyle	Crest
	Lateral condyle	Medial malleolus
	Tibial plateau	

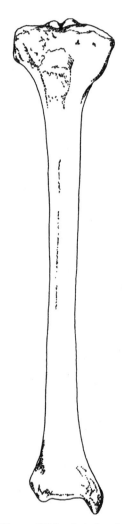

Figure 10.1 *Anterior view.*

FIBULA   Head   Lateral malleolus

TIBIA

FEMUR

PATELLA   Articular surface

CALCANEUS

KNEE JOINT

ANKLE JOINT

PATELLOFEMORAL JOINT

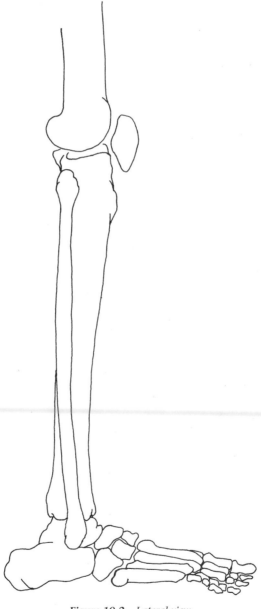

Figure 10.2   *Lateral view.*

B. Draw the major ligaments indicated above the drawings.

POSTERIOR CRUCIATE LIGAMENT

ANTERIOR CRUCIATE LIGAMENT

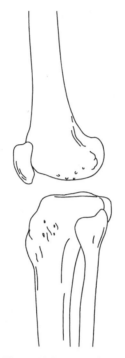

Figure 10.3   Lateral view.

LATERAL COLLATERAL LIGAMENT

LATERAL MENISCUS

MEDIAL COLLATERAL LIGAMENT

MEDIAL MENISCUS

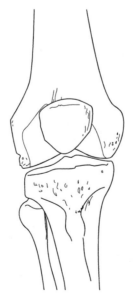

Figure 10.4   Anterior view.

2. On the drawings,

    A. Label the origin and insertion of the muscles listed.
       Color the origin in red and the insertion in blue.

    B. Join the origin and insertion to show the line of pull of the muscle.

    C. Review the hip lab for the hamstring muscles, adductors, and tensor fascia latae.

VASTUS LATERALIS

RECTUS FEMORIS

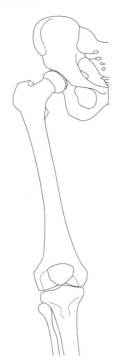 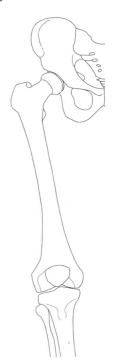

VASTUS MEDIALIS

VASTUS INTERMEDIALIS

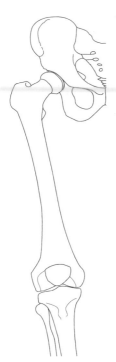 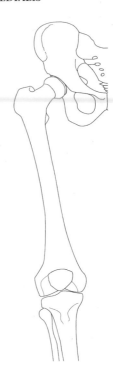

Figure 10.5   *Anterior view.*

POPLITEUS   GASTROCNEMIUS

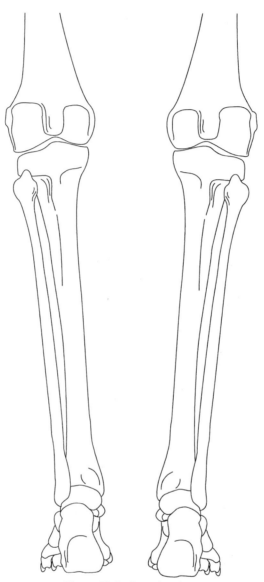

Figure 10.6   *Posterior view.*

3. For the knee joint, identify the following,

Shape	*Motion*	*Plane*	*Axis*

4. Name the structure of the knee joint that is concave. _____

   Name the structure of the knee joint that is convex. _____

5. Match each ligament and structure listed below with the appropriate function or characteristic. Each answer may be used more than once. Each function or characteristic may have more than one correct answer.

   _____ Posterior cruciate ligament

   _____ Anterior cruciate ligament

   _____ Lateral collateral ligament

   _____ Medial collateral ligament

   _____ Lateral meniscus

   _____ Medial meniscus

   A. Provides stability in the frontal plane
   B. Prevents anterior displacement of the tibia on the femur
   C. Fibers of the meniscus attach to this ligament
   D. Deepens the joint surface
   E. Prevents posterior displacement of the tibia on the femur
   F. Absorbs shock

6. For each motion listed, check the muscle(s) that are major contributors to that motion at the knee.

Motion	*Vastus lateralis*	*Vastus medialis*	*Vastus intermedialis*	*Rectus femoris*	*Semimem-branosus*	*Semiten-dinosus*	*Biceps femoris*	*Popliteus*	*Gastroc-nemius*
FLEXION									
EXTENSION									

7. Of the muscles listed in question 6,

   A. List those muscles that are multijoint muscles.

   B. Describe the position that simultaneously *lengthens* the multijoint muscle over all the joints it crosses.

Muscle	*Hip*	*Knee*	*Ankle*

8. Of the muscles listed in question 6,

    A. List those muscles that are single joint muscles.

    B. Describe each muscle's relationship to the knee—anterior or posterior.

    C. Describe the joint position that lengthens the muscle.

Muscle	Joint Surface	Lengthened Position

9. The sciatic nerve comes off which nerve roots? _____

    It descends down which side of the thigh? _____

    At the knee the sciatic nerve divides into two nerves. They are: _____

    _____

10. Describe the general pathway of the two divisions of the sciatic nerve as they descend to the foot.

    _____

    _____

    _____

11. Describe the general pathway of the femoral nerve and then identify the knee muscles it innervates. _____

    _____

12. During weight-bearing knee extension, in which direction does the femur rotate on the tibia during terminal extension? _____

13. During an open kinetic chain knee extension activity, in which direction does the tibia rotate on the femur to achieve terminal extension? _____

14. What is the Q angle? _____

    _____

15. What is the average Q angle? _____

LAB ACTIVITIES
KNEE JOINT

1. For each of the motions available at the knee joint, estimate the degrees of motion available by checking the box that most closely describes that motion. (Do not use a goniometer.)

Motion	*0–45*	*46–90*	*91–135*	*136–180*
FLEXION				
HYPEREXTENSION				

2. On the skeleton, anatomical models, and at least one partner, locate, palpate, and observe the structures described below. The reference position is the anatomical position. Having pictures for reference is helpful when trying to find the structures. Not all structures can be palpated.

Tibia

Intercondylar eminence: A double-pointed prominence approximately centered on the proximal surface of the tibia. It extends into the intercondyloid fossa of the femur. It cannot be palpated.

Medial condyle or medial plateau: The proximal medial aspect of the tibia. The distal and medial borders are not well defined. Palpate below the joint space on the medial aspect.

Lateral condyle or lateral plateau: The proximal lateral aspect of the tibia. The distal and medial borders are not well defined. Palpate below the joint space on the lateral aspect.

Tibial plateau: The broad proximal end of the tibia including the medial and lateral condyles or plateaus and the intercondylar eminence.

Tibial tuberosity: A protuberance in the midline of the anterior proximal surface of the tibia. Palpate the patella and move your fingers distal to the insertion of the patellar tendon on the tibial tuberosity.

Crest: The sharp anterior border of the shaft of the tibia. Palpate by moving your fingers distal from the tibial tuberosity along the ridge or crest.

Medial malleolus: Enlarged distal end of the tibia. Palpate on the medial aspect of the ankle.

Fibula

Head: The enlarged proximal end of the fibula. Palpate just below and slightly posterior to the lateral tibial condyle.

Lateral malleolus: The enlarged distal end of the fibula. Palpate on the lateral aspect of the ankle.

Patella: A triangular-shaped sesamoid bone on the anterior aspect of the knee. Palpate it on the anterior surface of the knee.

Other Structures

Posterior cruciate ligament: Located deep within the knee, it attaches to the tibia posteriorly in the intercondylar area and runs in a superior and anterior direction to attach anteriorly on the medial condyle of the femur. It cannot be palpated.

Anterior cruciate ligament: Located deep within the knee, it attaches to the tibia anteriorly in the intercondylar area and runs in a superior and posterior direction to attach posteriorly on the lateral condyle of the femur. It cannot be palpated.

Lateral collateral ligament: Located on the lateral aspect of the knee. It is a cordlike structure that spans the joint. The proximal attachment is the lateral condyle of the femur. The distal attachment is on the head of the fibula. With the knee extended, palpate on the lateral aspect of the knee by moving your finger perpendicular to the weight-bearing surface of the tibia.

Medial collateral ligament: Located on the medial aspect of the knee. It is a flat, broad ligament attaching proximally to the medial condyle of the femur and distally to the medial tibial condyle. The fibers of the medial meniscus attach to this ligament. It is not as easily palpated as the lateral collateral ligament.

Lateral meniscus: Located deep within the knee on the weight-bearing surface of the lateral tibial condyle. It cannot be palpated.

Medial meniscus: Located deep within the knee on the weight-bearing surface of the medial tibial condyle. It cannot be palpated.

3. Locate the muscles listed below on the skeleton, anatomical models, and at least one partner.

A. Locate the origin and insertion of the muscle on the skeleton.

B. Stretch a large rubber band taut by placing one end at the origin and the other end at the insertion of the muscle on the skeleton.

C. Perform the motion that muscle does and observe how the rubber band becomes less taut and shorter, similar to the muscle shortening as it contracts.

D. Perform the opposite motion and observe how the rubber band becomes more taut and longer, similar to the muscle lengthening as it is stretched.

E. After locating the muscle on the skeleton, locate the muscle on your partner. The position described for locating the muscle on your partner is the manual muscle test position for a fair or better grade of muscle strength. Not all origins, insertions, and muscle bellies can be palpated.

F. When possible, palpate the origin, insertion, and muscle belly of each muscle by:

1) Placing your fingers on the origin and insertion and asking your partner to contract the muscle.

2) Moving your fingers from the origin to the insertion over the contracting muscle.

3) Asking your partner to relax the muscle and again moving your fingers from the origin to the insertion over the muscle.

SITTING ON THE SIDE OF A TREATMENT TABLE (SHORT SITTING)

Rectus femoris: Located superficially on the anterior of the thigh.

Origin:	Anterior inferior iliac spine.
Insertion:	Tibial tuberosity via the patella tendon.
Action:	Extend the knee.
Palpate:	The midline of the quadriceps muscle or the patellar tendon.

Vastus lateralis: Located superficially and on the anterior lateral thigh.

Origin:	Linea aspera of the femur and greater trochanter.
Insertion:	Tibial tuberosity via the patella tendon.
Action:	Extend the knee.
Palpate:	The lateral portion of the quadriceps muscle or the patellar tendon.

Vastus medialis: Located superficially and on the anterior medial thigh.

Origin:	Linea aspera of the femur.
Insertion:	Tibial tuberosity via the patellar tendon.
Action:	Extend the knee.
Palpate:	The medial portion of the quadriceps muscle or the patellar tendon.

Vastus intermedialis: Located deep to the rectus femoris on the anterior thigh.

Origin:	Anterior femur.
Insertion:	Tibial tuberosity via the patellar tendon.
Action:	Extend the knee.
Palpate:	Difficult to palpate directly because it is deep to the rectus femoris.

PRONE POSITION

Semitendinosus: Located superficially on the posterior medial aspect of the thigh.

Position:	Prone with hip and knee extended.
Origin:	Ischial tuberosity.
Insertion:	Anteromedial surface of proximal tibia.
Action:	Flex the knee.
Palpate:	Superficially on the medial aspect of the posterior distal thigh just above the bend of the knee.

Semimembranosus: Located deep to the semitendinosus on the posterior medial thigh.

Position:	Prone with hip and knee extended.
Origin:	Ischial tuberosity.
Insertion:	Posterior surface of the medial plateau of the tibia.
Action:	Flex the knee.
Palpate:	On the medial aspect of the posterior distal thigh deep to, and on either side of, the semitendinosus tendon.

Biceps femoris: Located superficially on the posterior lateral aspect of the thigh just above the bend of the knee.

Position:	Prone with hip and knee extended.
Origin:	Long head: Ischial tuberosity Short head: Lateral lip of linea aspera.
Insertion:	Head of the fibula and lateral condyle of the tibia.
Action:	Flex the knee.
Palpate:	On the lateral aspect of the posterior distal thigh just above the bend of the knee.

Popliteus: Located deep to the gastrocnemius on the posterior proximal leg.

Position:	Prone with hip and knee extended.
Origin:	Lateral condyle of the femur.
Insertion:	On the posterior surface of the medial condyle of the tibia.
Action:	Flex the knee.
Palpate:	It is deep to the gastrocnemius and cannot be palpated.

STANDING POSITION

Gastrocnemius: Located superficially on the posterior of the leg.

Position:	Hip and knee extended.
Origin:	Posterior aspect of the medial and lateral condyles of the femur.
Insertion:	Via a common tendon onto the posterior aspect of the calcaneus.
Action:	Rise up on toes of the leg being observed.
Palpate:	On the posterior proximal medial and lateral aspects of the leg.

4. Use a disarticulated skeleton or anatomical model of the knee joint, and apply the rules of joint arthrokinematics and the concave-convex rule to perform the following exercises.

   A. Flex and extend the distal bone of the joint, the tibia, on the proximal bone, the femur. This is an open kinetic chain activity.

   B. Observe the movements of the tibia on the femur and circle the motions that you observed.

      Spin   Roll   Glide   None

   C. Again move the tibia on the femur and observe the movement of the tibia. Does the proximal end of the tibia move in the same or in the opposite direction as the distal end? _____

   _____

   D. Move the proximal bone of the joint, the femur, on the distal bone, the tibia, and observe the movement of the femur on the tibia. This is the motion that occurs in a closed kinetic chain activity.

   E. Circle the motions that you observed.

      Spin   Roll   Glide   None

   F. Again move the femur on the tibia. Did you observe the movement of the proximal end of the femur to be in the same or in the opposite direction as the distal end? _____

   _____

5. Referring to Worksheet question 7, assume the positions that make the multijoint muscles shorten simultaneously over all the joints they cross. Assume the positions that make the multijoint up muscles lengthen simultaneously over all the joints they cross.

6. With your partner prone and the knee fully flexed, perform a break test of the knee flexors. Note that this may cause a muscle cramp if you hold it for too long. Repeat with your partner supine with the hip and knee both fully flexed. Does the position of the hip, either flexed or extended, affect the strength of the hamstrings as knee flexors? _____

   Why? _____

   _____

7. *Varus* is described as the distal segment of a joint angled toward the midline. *Valgus* is described as the distal segment of a joint angled away from the midline. Varus or valgus at one joint may affect the alignment of other joints in a limb segment. The measurement of varus and valgus is based on the anatomical axis of one bone or bone segment in relation to the anatomical axis of another bone or bone segment comprising the joint.

   The anatomical axis is a line that runs along the shaft of a bone. The femur's anatomical axis is directed inferiorly and medially from proximal to distal. The anatomical axis of the tibia is directed almost vertically. The anatomical axes of the femur and tibia form an angle in the frontal plane that is measured at the lateral aspect of the knee with the axis at the knee joint. Normally the angle is 165 to 180 degrees and is described as slight genu valgus. *Genu* is another word for knee. *Genu valgus* is a pathological state with the femoral tibial angle of less than 165 degrees. This posture is commonly called "knock-knees." *Genu varus* is a pathological state with the femoral tibial angle of greater than 180 degrees. This posture is commonly called "bowlegs."

The hip angle to determine varus and valgus is the angle formed by the joining of the neck of the femur to the shaft of the femur. The normal angle for an adult is 125 degrees. *Coxa* is another word for hip. *Coxa varus* is the condition in which the angle of the femoral neck to the femoral shaft is less than 125 degrees. When coxa varus occurs, it is as if the femur must be adducted to place the head of the femur in the acetabulum. *Coxa valgus* is the condition in which the angle of the neck to the shaft is greater than 125 degrees. When coxa valgus occurs, it is as if the femur must be abducted to place the head of the femur in the acetabulum. Coxa varus often results in genu valgus. Coxa valgus may cause genu varus.

A. Observe your partners from a front view to determine whether genu valgus and genu varus are present.

B. Are the angles of the right and left lower extremities equal? _____

C. How many of your partner's angles are:

Within normal limits _____ Genu valgus _____ Genu varus _____

D. The knee generally has a few degrees of motion in the sagittal plane beyond 0 degrees of extension. This motion is hyperextension. *Genu recurvatum* is a pathological state of excessive knee hyperextension and is commonly called "back knee." Starting in the long sitting position, ask your partner to extend the knee as much as possible. Does the heel come off

the table and if so, how far? _____

With your partner standing, observe your partner from a lateral view to determine whether genu recurvatum is present.

8. What might be some of the effects on the weight-bearing surfaces of the knee when, because of varus, valgus, or recurvatum, the line of gravity does not fall in the normal position through the

knee joint? _____

_____

9. Diagram the lever that describes the activity at the knee joint when, starting in the standing position, a shallow knee bend is performed. *Analyze the down motion.*

A. On the figure, label the Xs that represent the axis, muscle, and gravity, and identify the specific joint and muscle group.

B. Make arrows out of the vertical lines to indicate the direction of the movement, the direction of the pull of the muscle, and the direction of gravity.

C. Identify the muscle and gravity as either *force* or *resistance*.

X	X	X	Direction of movement

10. Analyze the activity of the knee joint diagrammed in question No. 9 by answering the following questions.

   A. Which joint motion is being analyzed?_____

   B. Identify the "axis" of the motion._____

   C. Is the "force" producing the movement a muscle or gravity? _____

   D. Is the "resistance" to the movement a muscle or gravity? _____

   E. Which major muscle group is the agonist?_____

   F. Which major muscle group is the antagonist?_____

   G. Is the muscle acting to overcome gravity or slow down gravity? _____

   H. Is the agonist performing a concentric or an eccentric contraction?_____

   I. Is this an open or closed kinetic chain activity? _____

11. Diagram the lever that describes the activity at the knee joint during the activity of *returning to standing* from a shallow knee bend.

   A. On the figure, label the Xs that represent the axis, muscle, and gravity, and identify the specific joint and muscle group.

   B. Make arrows out of the vertical lines to indicate the direction of the movement, the direction of the pull of the muscle, and the direction of gravity.

   C. Identify the muscle and gravity as either *force* or *resistance*.

   X   X   X   Direction of movement

12. Analyze the activity of the knee joint diagrammed in question 11 by answering the following questions.

   A. Which joint motion is being analyzed?_____

   B. Identify the "axis" of the motion._____

   C. Is the "force" producing the movement a muscle or gravity? _____

   D. Is the "resistance" to the movement a muscle or gravity? _____

   E. Which major muscle group is the agonist?_____

   F. Which major muscle group is the antagonist?_____

   G. Is the muscle acting to overcome gravity or slow down gravity? _____

   H. Is the agonist performing a concentric or an eccentric contraction?_____

   I. Is this an open or closed kinetic chain activity? _____

13. Diagram the lever that describes the activity at the knee joint when, in the sitting position, the *knee is straightened against resistance.*

   A. On the figure, label the Xs that represent the axis, muscle, and gravity, and identify the specific joint and muscle group.

   B. Make arrows out of the vertical lines to indicate the direction of the movement, the direction of the pull of the muscle, and the direction of gravity.

   C. Identify the muscle and gravity as either *force* or *resistance.*

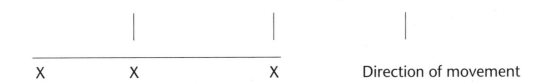

   X　　　　X　　　　　X　　　　Direction of movement

14. Analyze the activity of the knee joint diagrammed in question 13 by answering the following questions.

   A. Which joint motion is being analyzed?_____

   B. Is the movement moving with gravity or against gravity? _____

   C. Is there any external force giving resistance to the extremity? _____

   D. Which major muscle group is the agonist?_____

   E. Which major muscle group is the antagonist?_____

   F. Is the agonist performing a concentric or an eccentric contraction?_____

   G. Is this an open or closed kinetic chain activity? _____

15. Diagram the lever that describes the activity at the knee joint when, in the sitting position, the *knee is bent against resistance.*

   A. On the figure, label the Xs that represent the axis, muscle, and gravity, and identify the specific joint and muscle group.

   B. Make arrows out of the vertical lines to indicate the direction of the movement, the direction of the pull of the muscle, and the direction of gravity.

   C. Identify the muscle as either *force* or *resistance.*

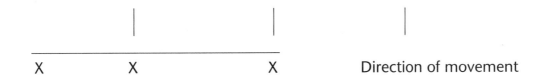

   X　　　　X　　　　　X　　　　Direction of movement

16. Analyze the activity of the knee joint diagrammed in question 15 by answering the following questions.

  A. Which joint motion is being analyzed?_____

  B. Is the movement moving with gravity or against gravity? _____

  C. Is there any external force giving resistance to the extremity? _____

  D. Which major muscle group is the agonist?_____

  E. Which major muscle group is the antagonist?_____

  F. Is the agonist performing a concentric or an eccentric contraction?_____

  G. Is this an open or closed kinetic chain activity? _____

17. Diagram the lever that describes the activity at the knee joint when, in the sidelying position, the *foot is moved toward the buttocks.*

  A. On the figure, label the Xs that represent the axis, muscle, and gravity, and identify the specific joint and muscle group.

  B. Make arrows out of the vertical lines to indicate the direction of the movement, the direction of the pull of the muscle, and the direction of gravity.

  C. Identify the muscle as either *force* or *resistance.*

```
        |              |                  |
  _____|__
   X          X              X          Direction of movement
```

18. Analyze the activity of the knee joint diagrammed in question 17 by answering the following questions.

  A. Which joint motion is being analyzed?_____

  B. What is the effect of gravity upon the movement? _____

  C. Is there any external force giving resistance to the extremity? _____

  D. Which major muscle group is the agonist?_____

  E. Which major muscle group is the antagonist?_____

  F. Is the agonist performing a concentric or an eccentric contraction?_____

  G. Is this an open or closed kinetic chain activity? _____

19. Diagram the lever that describes the activity at the knee joint when, in the sidelying position, the *foot is moved away from the buttocks*.

    A. On the figure, label the Xs that represent the axis, muscle, and gravity, and identify the specific joint and muscle group.

    B. Make arrows out of the vertical lines to indicate the direction of the movement, the direction of the pull of the muscle, and the direction of gravity.

    C. Identify the muscle as either *force* or *resistance*.

    |
          |
    _____ |
      X   X   X   Direction of movement

20. Analyze the activity of the knee joint diagrammed in question 19 by answering the following questions.

    A. Which joint motion is being analyzed?_____

    B. What is the effect of gravity upon the movement? _____

    C. Is there any external force giving resistance to the extremity? _____

    D. Which major muscle group is the agonist?_____

    E. Which major muscle group is the antagonist?_____

    F. Is the agonist performing a concentric or an eccentric contraction?_____

    G. Is this an open or closed kinetic chain activity? _____

POST-LAB QUESTIONS
KNEE JOINT

After you have completed the Worksheets and Lab Activities, answer the following questions without using your books or notes. When finished, check your answers.

1. You are working with a patient with a knee problem and are thinking about the muscles that cross the knee joint. Which muscle(s) that attach distally to the knee joint also attach proximally to the

   pelvis? _____

   _____

2. You are observing a patient who is post–cast removal for a fractured tibia. He cannot fully extend his knee. You are reviewing the muscles around the knee. Which muscle(s) that attach proximally

   to the knee also attach to the calcaneus?_____

   _____

3. A. Which muscles make up the hamstring muscle group?_____

   _____

   B. Which muscles make up the quadriceps muscle group? _____

   _____

   C. Which muscle(s) of the hamstring group do(es) not cross the hip joint?_____

   _____

   D. Which muscle of the quadriceps group does cross the hip joint?_____

   _____

4. Starting at the tibial tuberosity and proceeding laterally around the knee, name, in order, the muscles that span the knee joint._____

   _____

   _____

5. In which position is the hamstring group actively insufficient? _____

   In which position is the hamstring group passively insufficient? _____

6. In which position is the rectus femoris muscle actively insufficient?_____

   In which position is the rectus femoris muscle passively insufficient? _____

7. Are the Q angles for men and women equal? _____

8. Identify the varus and valgus deformities at the hips and knees in the following illustrations.

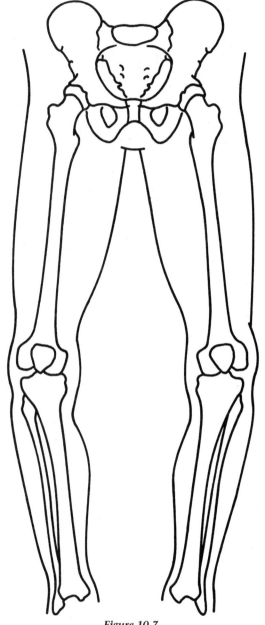

Figure 10.7

A. Coxa _____   B. Genu_____

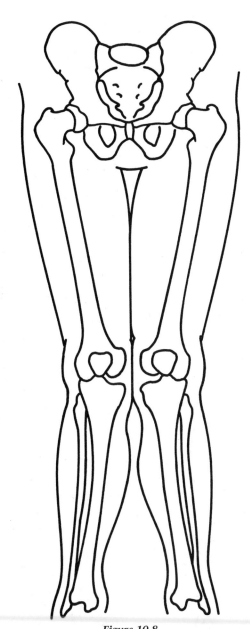

Figure 10.8

C. Coxa _____   D. Genu _____

9. Indicate the position (anterior, posterior, medial, or lateral) of the line of gravity to the center of the knee joint for the knee conditions listed below.

Line of Gravity

Knee Position	Anterior	Posterior	Medial	Lateral
VARUS				
VALGUS				
RECURVATUM				

10. Which muscles make up the *pes anserine* muscle group? _____

_____

11. A. Knee extensors are located on which side of the knee? _____

That muscle group is innervated by which nerve? _____

B. Knee flexors are located on which side of the knee? _____

12. Those knee flexors that also perform hip extension are called by what common name? _____

_____

That muscle group is innervated by which nerve? _____

13. What knee flexor is innervated by the common peroneal nerve? _____

Is it located on the medial or lateral side of the knee? _____

14. The popliteus muscle has its distal attachment on which side of the knee? _____

The popliteus muscle is innervated by which nerve? _____

11

ANKLE AND FOOT

Student's Name _____ Date Due _____

WORKSHEETS

Complete the following questions prior to lab class.

1. On the drawings, label the bones and major landmarks indicated.

TIBIA	Crest	Medial malleolus	Tuberosity
FIBULA	Head	Lateral malleolus	

OTHER STRUCTURES   Superior tibiofibular ligament and joint
Inferior tibiofibular ligament and joint
Interosseous membrane

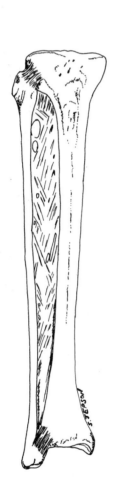
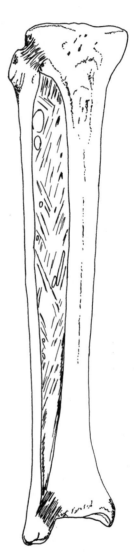

Figure 11.1   *Fibula and tibia.*

2. On the drawings,

A. Identify the view of the drawings.

B. Label the bones and landmarks of the foot.

(1) Calcaneus: Tuberosity   Sustentaculum tali
(2) Talus
(3) Navicular: Tuberosity
(4) Cuboid
(5) Cuneiforms: 1, 2, 3
(6) Metatarsals: 1, 2, 3, 4, 5:   Base   Head
(7) Phalanges: 1, 2, 3, 4, 5:   Proximal   Middle   Distal

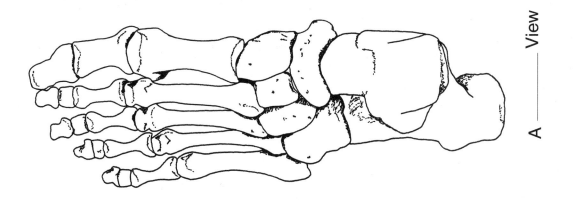

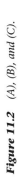

B _____ View

C _____ View

A _____ View

Figure 11.2 *(A), (B), and (C).*

3. On the drawings, label the joints and identify the bones of each joint.

   ANKLE JOINT

   SUBTALAR JOINT

   TRANSVERSE TARSAL JOINT

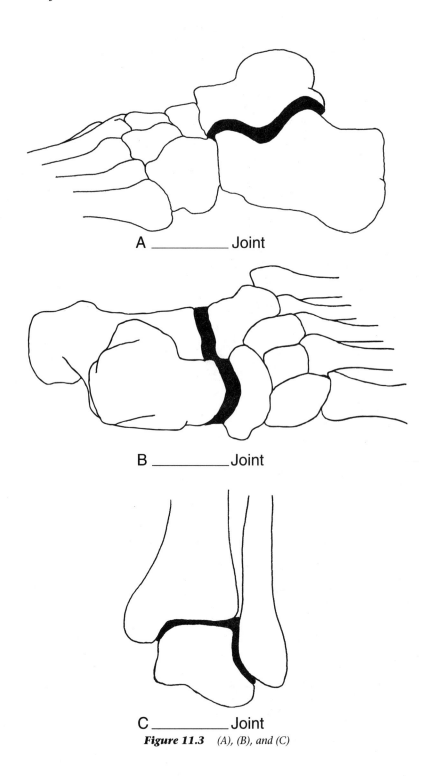

A _____ Joint

B _____ Joint

C _____ Joint

Figure 11.3   *(A), (B), and (C)*

METATARSAL PHALANGEAL JOINT

PROXIMAL INTERPHALANGEAL JOINT

DISTAL INTERPHALANGEAL JOINT

INTERPHALANGEAL JOINT

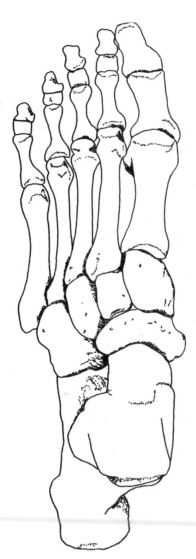

Figure 11.4

4. Identify the bones and label the ligaments on the drawings.

BONES	Tibia	Fibula	Cuboid	Metatarsals: 1–5
	Talus	Calcaneus	Cuneiforms: 1,2,3	

LIGAMENTS
Deltoid ligament
Inferior tibiofibular ligament
Lateral ligament
Long plantar ligament
Short plantar ligament
Spring ligament
Plantar aponeurosis

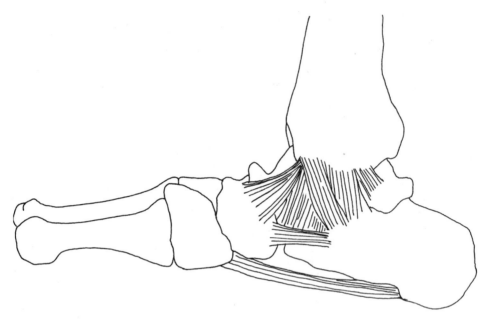

Figure 11.5 *Medial view. (Adapted from Kessler, RM, and Hertling, D: Management of Common Musculoskeletal Disorders. J B Lippincott, Philadelphia, 1983, p 457.)*

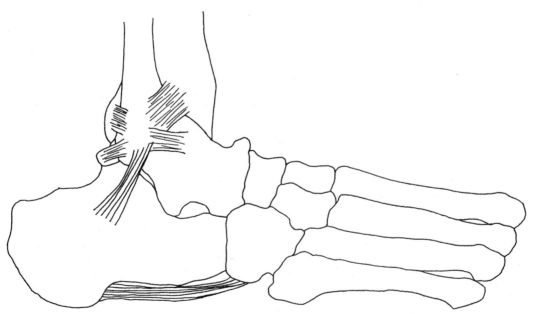

Figure 11.6 *Lateral view. (Adapted from Kessler, RM, and Hertling, D: Management of Common Musculoskeletal Disorders. J B Lippincott, Philadelphia, 1983, p 455.)*

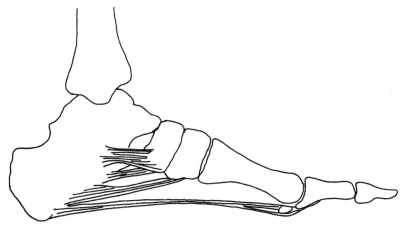

Figure 11.7   *Medial view.*

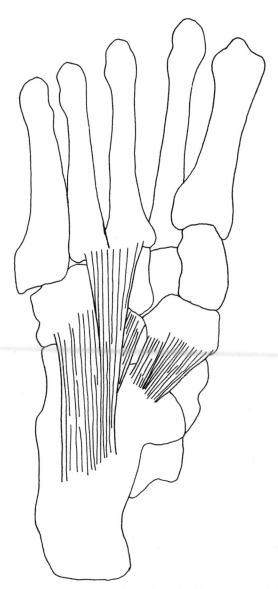

Figure 11.8   *Inferior view. (Adapted from Kessler, RM, and Hertling, D: Management of Common Musculoskeletal Disorders. J B Lippincott, Philadelphia, 1983, p 454.)*

5. On the drawings,

   A. Label the origin and insertion of the muscles listed.
      Color the origin in red and the insertion in blue.

   B. Join the origin and insertion to show the muscle belly.

   Gastrocnemius   Soleus   Plantaris

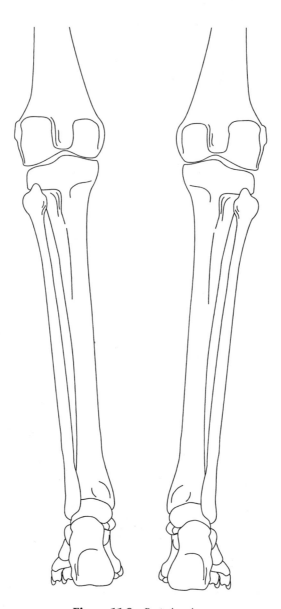

Figure 11.9 *Posterior view.*

Tibialis posterior

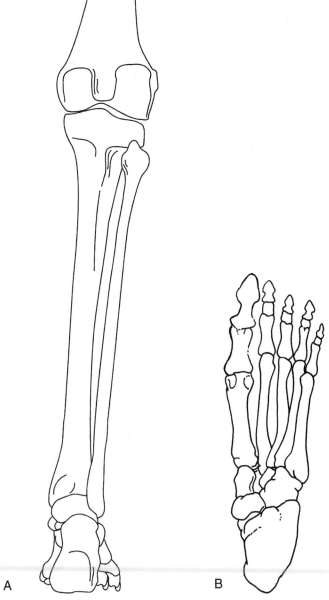

A   B

Figure 11.10 *(A) Posterior view. (B) Plantar view.*

Flexor hallucis longus

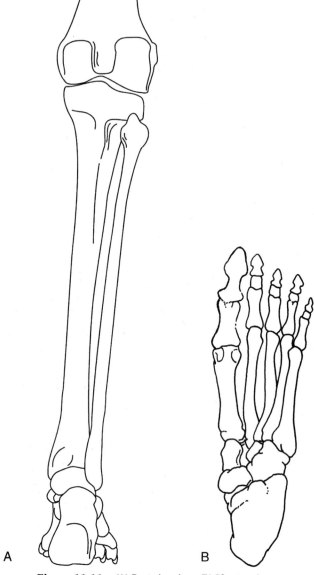

A   B

Figure 11.11   *(A) Posterior view. (B) Plantar view.*

Flexor digitorum longus

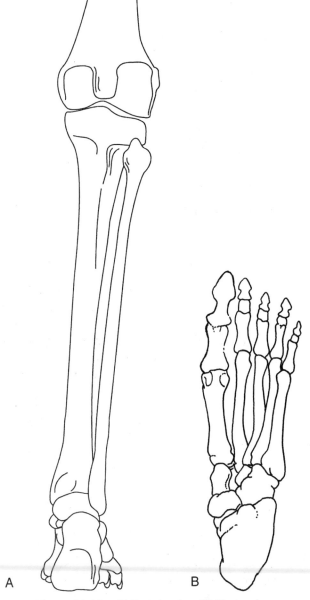

A   B

Figure 11.12   *(A) Posterior view. (B) Plantar view.*

Tibialis anterior   Extensor hallucis longus

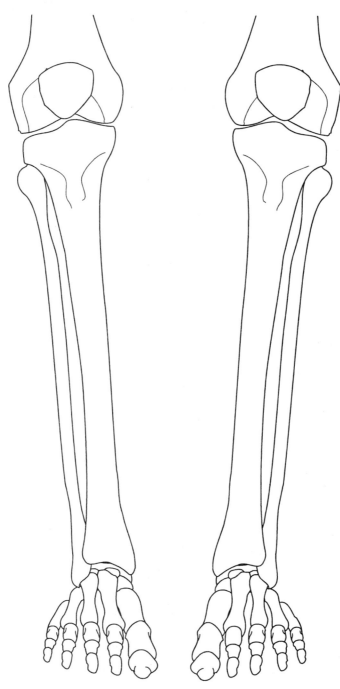

Figure 11.13 *Anterior view.*

Extensor digitorum longus

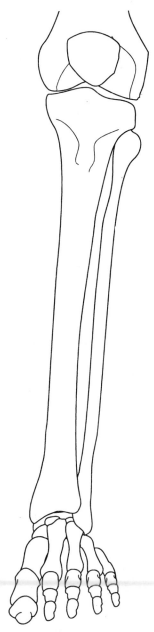

Figure 11.14 *Anterior view.*

Peroneus longus

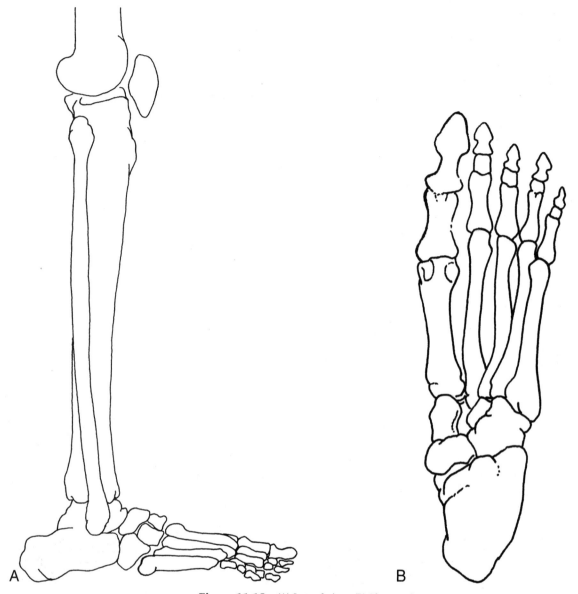

Figure 11.15 *(A) Lateral view. (B) Plantar view.*

Peroneus tertius

Peroneus brevis

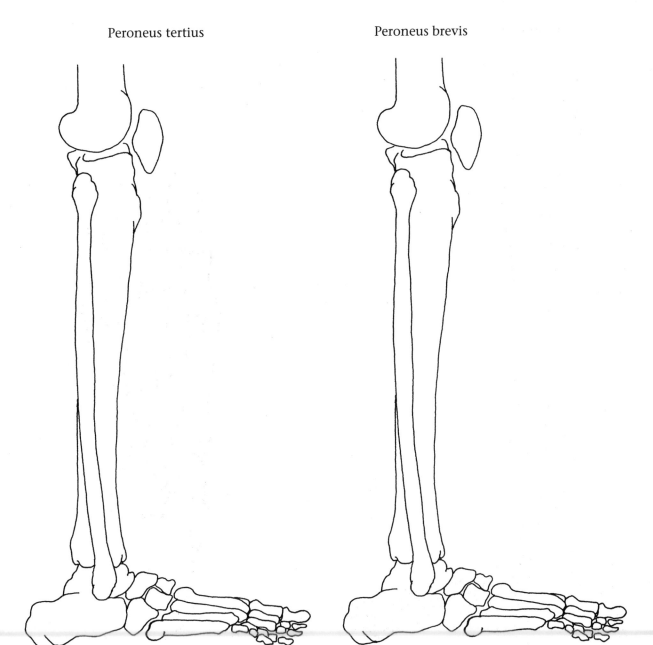

Figure 11.15 (Continued)

6. For each joint listed, identify the following.

Joint	Shape	Motions
Ankle (talocrural)		
Subtalar and transverse tarsal		
Metatarsal phalangeal		

7. List the bones that make up each of the following joints.

Ankle: _____

Subtalar: _____

Transverse tarsal: _____

Metatarsal phalangeal: _____

8. Match each ligament and structure listed below with the appropriate function or characteristic. Use each answer once.

_____ Deltoid ligament

_____ Medial longitudinal arch

_____ Spring ligament

_____ Plantar aponeurosis

_____ Transverse arch

_____ Lateral ligament

A. Three parts, each with one insertion on the fibula
B. Located on medial side and triangular in shape
C. Runs from side to side at the distal row of tarsals
D. Supports the medial side of the longitudinal arch
E. The talus is the keystone
F. Supports the longitudinal arch

9. For each motion listed, check the muscle(s) that are major contributors to that motion.

Ankle Motion	Gastrocnemius	Soleus	Plantaris	Tibialis posterior	Flexor hallucis longus	Flexor digitorum longus	Tibialis anterior	Extensor hallucis longus	Extensor digitorum longus	Peroneus longus	Peroneus brevis	Peroneus tertius
PLANTAR FLEXION												
DORSIFLEXION												
EVERSION												
INVERSION												

Toe(s) Motion	Extensor digitorum brevis	Flexor hallucis longus	Flexor digitorum longus	Extensor hallucis longus	Extensor digitorum longus	Abductor hallucis	Flexor digitorum brevis	Abductor digiti minimi	Quadratus plantae	Lumbricales	Flexor hallucis brevis	Adductor hallucis	Flexor digiti inimi	Dorsal interossei	Plantar interossei
FLEXION															
EXTENSION															
ABDUCTION															
ADDUCTION															

227

10. Of the muscles listed in question 9 except the intrinsics of the foot,

   A. List those muscles that are multijoint muscles.

   B. Describe the position that simultaneously *lengthens* the multijoint muscle over each joint it passes.

Muscle	Knee	Ankle	Foot (subtalar and transverse tarsal)	MP	IP

11. Diagram the lever that describes the activity at the ankle joint during the *lowering phase of a squat.*

    A. On the figure, label the Xs that represent the axis, muscle, and gravity, and identify the specific joint and muscle group.

    B. Make arrows out of the vertical lines to indicate the direction of the movement, the direction of the pull of the muscle, and the direction of the gravity.

    C. Identify the muscle and gravity as either *force* or *resistance*.

    X   X   X   Direction of movement

12. Analyze the activity at the ankle joint diagrammed in question 11 by answering the following questions.

    A. Which joint motion is being analyzed? _____

    B. Identify the "axis" of the motion. _____

    C. Is the "force" producing the movement a muscle or gravity? _____

    D. Is the "resistance" to the movement a muscle or gravity? _____

    E. Which major muscle group is the agonist? _____

    F. Which major muscle group is the antagonist? _____

    G. Is the muscle acting to overcome or slow down gravity? _____

    H. Is the agonist performing a concentric or an eccentric contraction? _____

    I. Is this an open or closed kinetic chain activity? _____

13. Diagram the lever that describes the activity at the ankle joint during the *rising phase of a squat*.

   A. On the figure, label the Xs that represent the axis, muscle, and gravity, and identify the specific joint and muscle group.

   B. Make arrows out of the vertical lines to indicate the direction of the movement, the direction of the pull of the muscle, and the direction of gravity.

   C. Identify the muscle and gravity as either *force* or *resistance*.

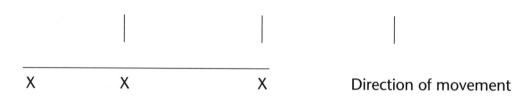

X   X   X   Direction of movement

14. Analyze the activity at the ankle joint diagrammed in question 13 by answering the following questions.

   A. Which joint motion is being analyzed?_____

   B. Identify the "axis" of the motion._____

   C. Is the "force" producing the movement a muscle or gravity? _____

   D. Is the "resistance" to the movement a muscle or gravity? _____

   E. Which major muscle group is the agonist?_____

   F. Which major muscle group is the antagonist?_____

   G. Is the muscle acting to overcome or slow down gravity? _____

   H. Is the agonist performing a concentric or an eccentric contraction?_____

   I. Is this an open or closed kinetic chain activity? _____

LAB ACTIVITIES
ANKLE AND FOOT

1. For each of the motions listed, estimate the degrees of motion available by checking the box that most closely describes that motion. (Do not use a goniometer.)

Motion	0–45	46–90	91–135	136–180
DORSIFLEXION				
PLANTAR FLEXION				
INVERSION				
EVERSION				

2. On the skeleton, anatomical models, and at least one partner, locate, palpate, and observe the structures described below. The reference position is the anatomical position. Having pictures for reference is helpful when trying to find the structures. Not all structures can be palpated.

Tibia: See the lab chapter on the knee for other landmarks of the tibia.

Crest: The anterior prominent border. Palpate along the front of the leg.

Medial malleolus: The enlarged distal medial surface. Palpate on the medial side of the ankle.

Fibula: The lateral bone of the leg.

Head: The enlarged proximal end. Palpate below the knee joint on the lateral side of the leg.

Lateral malleolus: The enlarged distal end. Palpate on the lateral side of the ankle.

Tarsals

Calcaneus: The largest and most posterior tarsal bone. Palpate by grasping the heel.

Sustentaculum tali: A small protuberance on the medial superior part of the calcaneus.

Talus: Articulates with the tibia to form the ankle joint.

Navicular: Located on the medial side anterior to the talus and proximal to the cuneiforms.

Tuberosity: A protuberance on the medial aspect of the navicular. Palpate on the medial side of the foot below the medial malleolus.

Cuboid: Located on the lateral side of the foot between the calcaneus and the fourth and fifth metatarsals. Palpate on the lateral side of the foot just proximal to the metatarsals.

Cuneiforms: There are three cuneiforms. The first is located on the medial side of the foot, the second is lateral to the first, and the third is between the second cuneiform and the cuboid. The cuneiforms are distal to the navicular and proximal to the metatarsals. Palpate starting on the medial side of the foot.

Metatarsals: There are five metatarsals. Located between the cuneiforms, cuboid, and the phalanges. Palpate between the cuneiforms, cuboid, and phalanges each in turn starting on the medial and progressing laterally.

Base: The proximal end of a metatarsal.
Head: The distal end of a metatarsal.

Phalanges: The great toe has two phalanges and each of the remaining toes has three. The phalanges are described as the proximal, middle, or distal phalanges. Palpate distal to the metatarsal phalangeal joint.

3. Locate the muscles listed below on the skeleton and on at least one partner.

A. Locate the origin and insertion of the muscle on the skeleton.

B. Stretch a large rubber band taut by placing one end at the origin and the other end at the insertion of the muscle on the skeleton.

C. Perform the motion that muscle does and observe how the rubber band becomes less taut and shorter, similar to the muscle shortening as it contacts.

D. Perform the opposite motion and observe how the rubber band becomes more taut and longer, similar to the muscle lengthening as it is stretched.

E. After locating the muscle on the skeleton, locate the muscle on your partner. The position described for locating the muscle is the manual muscle test position for a fair or better grade of muscle strength. Not all origins, insertions, and muscle bellies can be palpated.

F. When possible, palpate the origin, insertion, and muscle belly of each muscle by:

1) Placing your fingers on the origin and insertion and asking your classmate to contract the muscle.

2) Moving your fingers from the origin to the insertion over the contracting muscle.

3) Asking your partner to relax the muscle and again moving your fingers from the origin to the insertion over the muscle belly.

STANDING POSITION

Gastrocnemius: Located superficially on the posterior leg.

Position:	Standing on the limb to be tested.
Origin:	Medial head: Medial condyle of femur.
	Lateral head: Lateral condyle of femur.
Insertion:	Posterior calcaneus.
Action:	Raise up on toes.
Palpate:	Posterior aspect of the leg.

Soleus: Located deep to the gastrocnemius muscle.

Position:	Standing on the limb to be tested with the knee slightly flexed. Individual may need support for balance.
Origin:	Posterior tibia and fibula.
Insertion:	Posterior calcaneus.
Action:	Raise up on toes.
Palpate:	Distally on the posterior aspect of the leg.

Plantaris: Located deep to the lateral head of the gastrocnemius muscle.

Position:	Standing on limb to be tested.
Origin:	Posterior lateral condyle of femur.
Insertion:	Posterior calcaneus.
Action:	Raise up on toes.
Palpate:	Because this muscle is small and deep to the gastrocnemius, it cannot be palpated.

SHORT SITTING (SITTING ON SIDE OF TREATMENT TABLE)

Tibialis Posterior: Located deep to the soleus and gastrocnemius.

Position:	Sitting with the foot not touching floor.
Origin:	Interosseous membrane and adjacent proximal tibia and fibula.
Insertion:	Navicular, calcaneus, and cuneiforms.
Action:	Invert the foot.
Palpate:	The tendon can be palpated above the medial malleolus and between the medial malleolus and navicular.

Flexor hallucis longus: Located deep to the soleus and gastrocnemius on the lateral aspect of the leg.

Position:	Sitting with the foot supported on the examiner's lap.
Origin:	Posterior fibula and interosseous membrane.
Insertion:	Base of the distal phalanx of the great toe.
Action:	Flex the great toe.
Palpate:	At the insertion and posterior to the medial malleolus.

Flexor digitorum longus: Located deep to the soleus and gastrocnemius on the medial aspect of the leg.

Position:	Sitting with the foot supported on the examiner's lap.
Origin:	Posterior tibia.
Insertion:	Base of the distal phalanges of the four lateral toes.
Action:	Flex the four lateral toes.
Palpate:	Posterior to the medial malleolus.

Tibialis anterior: Located superficially on the anterior lateral aspect of the leg.

Position:	Sitting with the foot supported on the examiner's lap.
Origin:	Lateral tibia and interosseous membrane.
Insertion:	First cuneiform and metatarsal.
Action:	Dorsiflex the ankle and invert the foot.
Palpate:	Palpate the belly on the lateral aspect of the tibia and the tendon on the anterior aspect of the ankle.

Extensor hallucis longus: Located deep to the tibialis anterior and extensor digitorum longus muscles.

Position:	Sitting with the foot supported on the examiner's lap.
Origin:	Fibula and interosseous membrane.
Insertion:	Dorsal on the distal phalanx of the great toe.
Action:	Extend the great toe.
Palpate:	Palpate the tendon on the dorsum of the foot.

Extensor digitorum longus: Located deep to the tibialis anterior on the anterior lateral aspect of the tibia.

Position:	Sitting with the foot supported on the examiner's lap.
Origin:	Fibula, interosseous membrane, and tibia.
Insertion:	Distal phalanges of the lateral four toes.
Action:	Extend the four lateral toes.
Palpate:	Palpate the tendons on the dorsum of the foot.

Peroneus longus: Partially covered by the tibialis anterior and superficial to the other peroneal muscles on the anterior lateral aspect of the leg.

Position:	Sitting with the ankle at neutral and the foot not touching the floor.
Origin:	Proximal fibula, lateral condyle of tibia, and interosseous membrane.
Insertion:	Plantar surface of the first cuneiform and metatarsal.
Action:	Evert the foot.
Palpate:	The muscle belly can be palpated distal to the head of the fibula. The tendon can be palpated posterior to the lateral malleolus and the peroneus brevis muscle.

Peroneus brevis: Located deep to the peroneus longus on the lateral aspect of the leg.

Position:	Sitting with the ankle at neutral and the foot not touching the floor.
Origin:	Lateral distal fibula.
Insertion:	Base of the fifth metatarsal.
Action:	Evert the foot.
Palpate:	The muscle belly can be palpated on the lower lateral aspect of the fibula. The tendon can be palpated from inferior to the lateral malleolus to its distal attachment.

Peroneus tertius: Located deep to the peroneus longus and the extensor digitorum longus on the anterior lateral aspect of the leg.

Position:	Sitting with the ankle at neutral and the foot not touching the floor.
Origin:	Distal medial fibula.
Insertion:	Dorsal surface of the base of the fifth metatarsal.
Action:	Evert the foot.
Palpate:	The tendon can be palpated from anterior to the lateral malleolus on the dorsum of the foot to its distal attachment.

Extensor digitorum brevis: Located superficially on the dorsum of the foot.

Position:	Sitting with the foot supported in the examiner's lap.
Origin:	Dorsal surface of the calcaneus.
Insertion:	On the proximal phalanx of the great toe and with the extensor digitorum longus of the four lateral toes.
Action:	Extend the toes.
Palpate:	On the dorsum of the foot.

Abductor hallucis: Located superficially on the medial aspect of the foot.

Position:	Sitting with the foot supported in the examiner's lap.
Origin:	Medial aspect of the calcaneus and plantar aponeurosis.
Insertion:	Medial side of the proximal phalanx of the great toe.
Action:	Abduct the great toe.
Palpate:	On the medial aspect of the foot.

Flexor digitorum brevis: Located deep to the plantar aponeurosis on the plantar surface of the foot.

Position:	Sitting with the foot supported in the examiner's lap.
Origin:	Calcaneus and plantar aponeurosis.
Insertion:	Both sides of the middle phalanges of the four lateral toes.
Action:	Flex the toes.
Palpate:	Cannot be palpated.

Abductor digiti minimi: Located superficially on the lateral aspect of the foot.

Position:	Sitting with the foot supported in the examiner's lap.
Origin:	Calcaneus and plantar aponeurosis.
Insertion:	Lateral aspect of the base of the proximal phalanx of the fifth toe.
Action:	Abduct the little toe.
Palpate:	On the lateral aspect of the foot.

Quadratus plantae: Located deep to the plantar aponeurosis on the sole of the foot.

Position:	Sitting with the foot supported in the examiner's lap.
Origin:	Calcaneus and long plantar ligament.
Insertion:	Tendon of the flexor digitorum longus.
Action:	Flex the four lateral toes.
Palpate:	Cannot be palpated.

Lumbricales: Located deep on the plantar surface of the foot.

Position:	Sitting with the foot supported in the examiner's lap.
Origin:	First: Medial aspect of the flexor digitorum longus tendon. Second, third, and fourth: Adjacent sides of the flexor digitorum longus tendons.
Insertion:	Proximal phalanges of the four lateral toes and tendons of the extensor digitorum longus.
Action:	Flex the MP joints and extend the PIP and DIP joints of the four lateral toes.
Palpate:	Cannot be palpated.

Flexor hallucis brevis: Located deep to the plantar aponeurosis on the plantar surface of the foot.

Position:	Sitting with the foot supported in the examiner's lap.
Origin:	Plantar surface of the calcaneus, cuboid, and tibialis posterior tendon.
Insertion:	Medial and lateral aspects of the proximal phalanx of the great toe.
Action:	Flex the MP joint of the great toe.
Palpate:	Cannot be palpated.

Adductor hallucis: Located deep to the plantar aponeurosis superficially on the medial aspect of the foot.

Position:	Sitting with the foot supported in the examiner's lap.
Origin:	Base of the second, third, and fourth metatarsal bones and adjacent ligaments.
Insertion:	Lateral sesamoid bone and base of the first phalanx of the great toe.
Action:	Adduct the great toe.
Palpate:	Cannot be palpated.

Flexor digiti minimi: Located deep to the plantar aponeurosis on the plantar surface of the foot.

Position:	Sitting with the foot supported in the examiner's lap.
Origin:	Plantar surface of the base of the fifth metatarsal.
Insertion:	Lateral aspect of the base of the proximal phalanx of the fifth toe.
Action:	Flex the MP joint of the fifth toe.
Palpate:	Cannot be palpated.

Dorsal interossei: Located deep to all structures on the dorsum of the foot.

Position:	Sitting with the foot supported in the examiner's lap.
Origin:	Adjacent sides of the metatarsal bone.
Insertion:	Tendons of the extensor digitorum longus of toes one through four.
Action:	Abduct toes two, three, and four.
Palpate:	Cannot be palpated.

Plantar interossei: Located deep to all structures on the plantar surface of the foot.

Position:	Sitting with the foot supported in the examiner's lap.
Origin:	Medial aspects of the base of the third, fourth, and fifth metatarsal bones.
Insertion:	Medial aspect of the base of the respective toe proximal phalanx.
Action:	Adduct and flex the MP joints of the lateral three toes.
Palpate:	Cannot be palpated.

4. Describe the positions of the malleoli in relation to one another. _____

_____

5. Does the position of the knee affect the range of motion available at the ankle? Explain. _____

_____

_____

6. A. In the short sitting position and in an open kinetic chain perform a concentric contraction and then an eccentric contraction of the tibialis anterior.

   When performing the concentric contraction, are the origin and insertion moving toward or

   away from each other? _____

   When performing the eccentric contraction, are the origin and insertion moving toward or

   away from each other? _____

   B. Stand with your back about 6 inches away from a wall. Lean backward from your ankles until your shoulders touch the wall. Return to standing erect. What type of contraction is the

   anterior tibialis performing as you lean back? _____

   Is the origin moving toward or away from the insertion?_____

   What type of contraction is the anterior tibialis performing as you return to standing? _____

   _____

   Is the origin moving toward or away from the insertion?_____

   C. What is the term used to describe the muscle action that occurs when the origin moves toward

   the insertion? _____

   Does this type of muscle action occur in an open or a closed kinetic chain activity?

   _____

7. Perform ankle dorsiflexion without using the anterior tibialis muscle. Which muscles can

   substitute for or assist the tibialis anterior muscle to dorsiflex the ankle? _____

   _____

8. The *anatomical axis* of the tibia and calcaneus normally forms only a very slight angle. The angle is measured by aligning the goniometer over the midline of the posterior tibia and midline of the posterior calcaneus with the axis at the ankle joint.

   Calcaneal varus is a decreased angle from the normal angle of the tibia and calcaneus. The calcaneus appears to be inverted.

   Calcaneal valgus is an increased angle from the normal angle of the tibia and calcaneus. The calcaneus appears to be everted.

   A. Observe your partner's tibial calcaneal angle in the standing position.

   Describe the position of the calcaneus in relation to the tibia. _____

   _____

   B. Are the angles equal? _____

   C. Observe the heels of your partner's shoes for the part of the heel that is most worn. Does

   this correlate with the position of the calcaneus?_____

9. Dip the sole of one foot in a tub of water and then briefly step on a paper towel. Observe the water mark your foot left on the paper towel.

   A. Describe the parts of your foot that contacted the supporting surface._____

   _____

   B. Compare your pattern of weight distribution to the normal. _____

   _____

10. Diagram the lever that describes the activity at the *right ankle when descending the stairs leading with your left foot*. Start facing down the stairs with both feet on the first step. Lower your left foot to the floor.

   A. On the figure, label the Xs that represent the axis, muscle, and gravity, and identify the specific joint and muscle group.

   B. Make arrows out of the vertical lines to indicate the direction of the movement, the direction of the pull of the muscle, and the direction of gravity.

   C. Identify the muscle and gravity as either *force* or *resistance*.

X	X	X	Direction of movement

11. Analyze the activity at the ankle joint diagrammed in question 10 by answering the following questions.

    A. Which joint motion is being analyzed?_____

    B. Identify the "axis" of the motion._____

    C. Is the "force" producing the movement a muscle or gravity? _____

    D. Is the "resistance" to the movement a muscle or gravity? _____

    E. Which major muscle group is the agonist?_____

    F. Which major muscle group is the antagonist?_____

    G. Is the muscle acting to overcome or slow down gravity? _____

    H. Is the agonist performing a concentric or an eccentric contraction? _____

    I. Is this an open or closed kinetic chain activity? _____

POST-LAB QUESTIONS
ANKLE AND FOOT

After you have completed the Worksheets and Lab Activities, answer the following questions without using your books or notes. When finished, check your answers.

1. List the motions that occur at the:

   A. Ankle joint. _____

   _____

   B. Subtalar joint. _____

   _____

   C. Transverse tarsal joint. _____

   _____

2. List the bones to which the deltoid ligament attaches. _____

   _____

3. What maintains the normal arches of the foot? _____

   _____

   _____

4. Why might a person have less ankle dorsiflexion when the knee is extended?_____

   _____

5. The proper names for the "Tom, Dick, and Harry" muscles are _____

   _____

   _____

   Identify the location where these muscles are in the order Tom, Dick, and Harry. _____

   _____

6. Indicate the relationship of the distal tendons of the peroneal muscles to the lateral malleolus.

   Peroneus longus _____

   Peroneus brevis _____

   Peroneus tertius _____

7. In general, which nerves innervate the muscles that:

   Dorsiflex _____

   Plantarflex _____

   Evert _____

8. What is the effect of toe extension on the longitudinal arch of the foot? _____

   _____

   _____

9. What position would the calcaneus assume when the following ligaments are ruptured?

   A. Lateral ligament: _____

   B. Deltoid ligament: _____

10. In the following examples, identify the type of isotonic contraction and the muscle(s) performing the contraction.

    A. In the standing position rising up on the toes. _____

    _____

    B. From standing on toes to lowering the foot back to the floor. _____

    _____

    C. Pushing on the gas pedal while driving a car. _____

    _____

11. Which muscle(s) attach on the base of the fifth metatarsal? _____

    _____

12. List the muscle(s) that cross the ankle posteriorly and have their primary action at the:

    A. Ankle. _____

    B. Foot. _____

    C. Toes. _____

13. Which muscle(s) attach to the femur and the calcaneus? _____

    _____

14. Starting at the anterior medial aspect of the ankle, name the extrinsic muscles and tendons that

    cross the ankle as you move laterally around the ankle joint. _____

    _____

    _____

15. Which muscle "straightens" the line of pull of the toe flexors? _____

    _____

16. The sustentaculum tali is located on which bone? _____

17. When an individual is unable to actively dorsiflex the ankle against gravity due to nerve damage, which nerve is damaged? _____

18. If the tibial nerve is damaged, which ankle motion would an individual not be able to actively perform? _____

19. Which muscles act as neutralizers to the extensor hallucis longus when in an open kinetic chain and only toe extension is desired? _____

_____

12

NECK, TRUNK, AND RESPIRATION

Introduction to the Vertebral Column

The joints and motions of the vertebral column are complex. The types of joints found in the vertebral column are described by their location. The anterior joints are referred to as the *intervertebral joints* and the posterior joints are called *facet joints*.

The anterior joints, the intervertebral joints, are located between adjacent vertebral bodies. These joints are amphiarthrodial and cartilaginous joints.

Each vertebra has two posterior joints, the facet joints, located between two adjacent vertebrae on either side of the spinous process. These joints are made up of the superior articular process of the vertebra below articulating with the inferior articular process of the vertebra above. These joints are described as *diathrodial, synovial,* and *plane joints*. Little motion occurs at each joint,

but in combination, all the joints of the vertebral column produce a significant amount of motion in all three planes.

Because of the direction of the facet joints at the three regions (cervical, thoracic, and lumbar) of the vertebral column, the amount of motion in the different planes varies. The cervical region has the most motion in all three planes. The thoracic region has rotation and lateral bending but little flexion and extension. The lumbar region has mostly flexion and extension with little rotation and lateral bending.

The first two cervical vertebrae are exceptions. The atlanto-occipital joint allows only flexion and extension, as in nodding "yes" with the head. The atlanto-axial joint allows only rotation as in shaking the head to indicate "no."

Introduction to the Pelvic Girdle

The position of the pelvis is determined in part by the major muscle groups attached to it. The orientation of the pelvis is identified by the position of the anterior superior iliac spines (ASIS) in relation to the pubic symphysis. When the ASIS is anterior to the pubic symphysis, the position of

the pelvis is labeled *anterior pelvic tilt* (Fig. 12.1). When the ASIS is posterior to the pubic symphysis, the position of the pelvis is labeled *posterior pelvic tilt* (Fig. 12.2). The anterior and posterior pelvic tilt is movement in the sagittal plane around the frontal axis. In the frontal plane, the iliac crests are normally level. When the iliac crests are uneven, the position is described as *lateral pelvic tilt* (Fig. 12.3), and the high side is identified; for example, lateral pelvic tilt to the right or *right lateral pelvic tilt*.

The abdominal muscles and the hamstring muscle group make up a force couple that produces a *posterior pelvic tilt* when the muscles contract concentrically. The trunk extensors and the

hip flexors acting together produce an *anterior pelvic tilt*. A *lateral pelvic tilt* is produced by the hip abductors of one side and the quadratus lumborum on the opposite side. In each position, one muscle group can usually produce the position, or the force couple acting together can produce the position. The normal resting position of the pelvis is a result of a balance between the force couples.

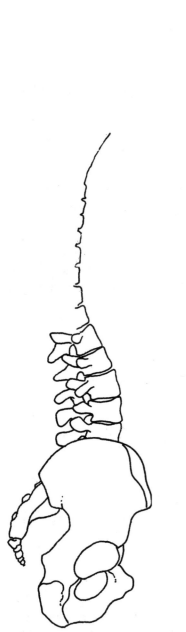

Figure 12.1 Anterior pelvic tilt.

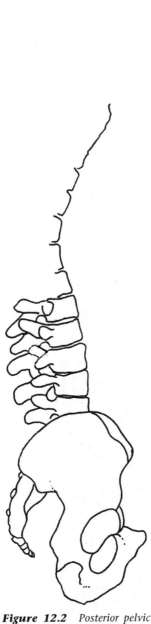

Figure 12.2 Posterior pelvic tilt.

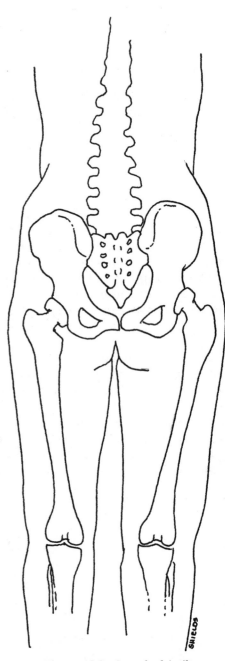

Figure 12.3 Lateral pelvic tilt.

WORKSHEETS
NECK, TRUNK, AND RESPIRATION

Complete the following questions prior to lab class.

1. **A.** Label the four regions of the vertebral column.

      Cervical spine   Thoracic spine
      Lumbar spine   Sacral spine

    B. Indicate which regions are:

      Concave (lordotic)   Convex (kyphotic)

    C. Identify:

      C7   T12   L5

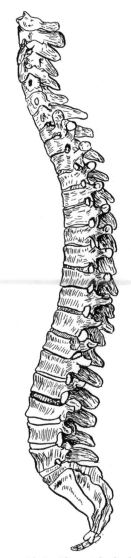

Figure 12.4   *The vertebral column.*

2. On the drawings, label the bones and major landmarks indicated.

SKULL   Occipital bone   Frontal bone   Temporal bone
                     Parietal bone   Mandible   Maxilla
                     Mastoid process

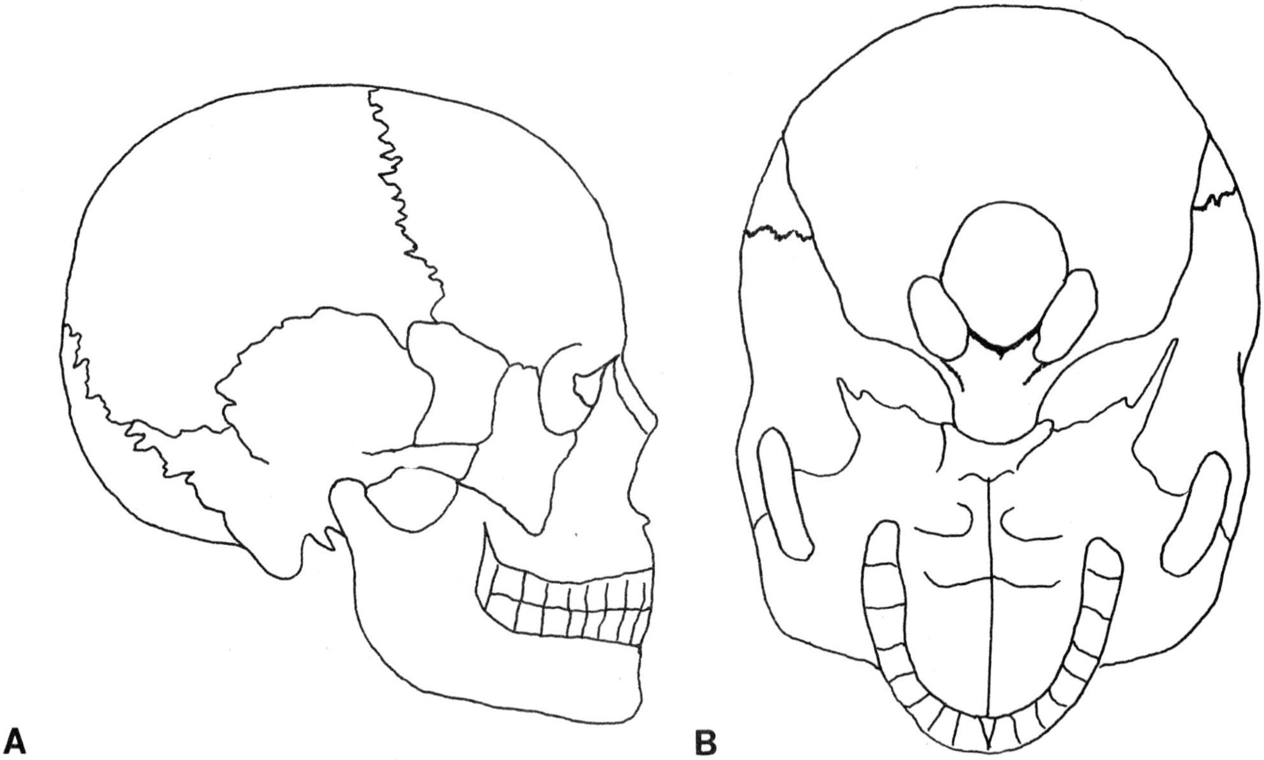

A   B

Figure 12.5 *(A) Lateral view. (B) Inferior view.*

VERTEBRA   Body   Neural arch   Vertebral foramen
                     Pedicle   Lamina   Transverse process
                     Spinous process   Articular process

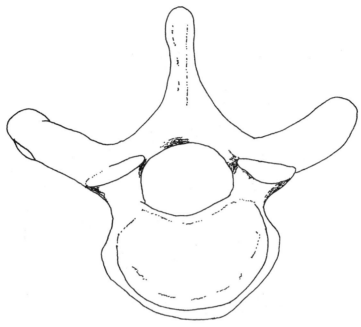

Figure 12.6 *Superior view.*

VERTEBRAE   Intervertebral foramen   Inferior articular process
                     Superior articular process

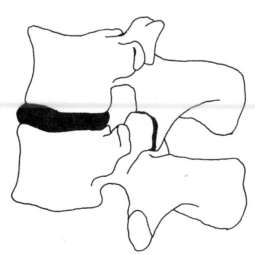

Figure 12.7 *Lateral view.*

ATLAS   Anterior arch   Articular process   **Transverse foramen**
                     Posterior arch   Transverse process   **Vertebral foramen**

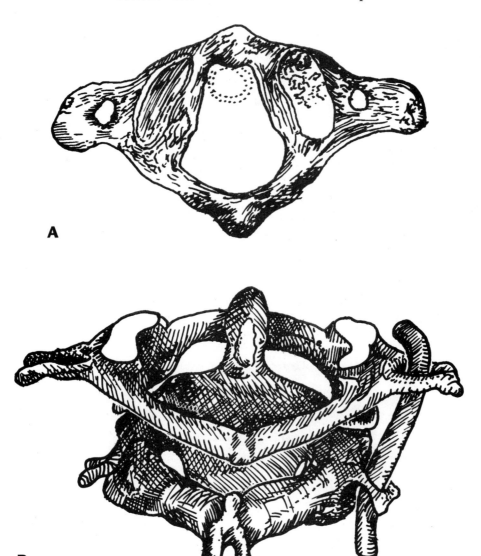

A

B

Figure 12.8   *(A) The atlas. (B) Atlas and axis. ([B] adapted from Norkin, CC, and Levangie, PK: Joint Structure and Function: A*
                     Comprehensive Analysis, ed 2. FA Davis, Philadelphia, 1992, p 146.)

AXIS   Dens (odontoid process)   Superior articular process
        Transverse foramen

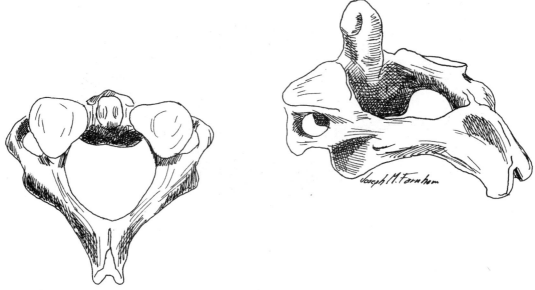

Figure 12.9   *The axis. (From Norkin, CC, and Levangie, PK: Joint Structure and Function: A Comprehensive Analysis, ed 2. FA Davis, Philadelphia, 1992, p 146, with permission.)*

INTERVERTEBRAL DISK   Annulus fibrosus   Nucleus pulposus

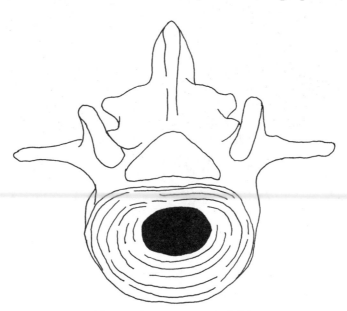

Figure 12.10   *Intervertebral disk.*

COSTAL FACET

DEMIFACET

VERTEBRAL BODY

Articular process

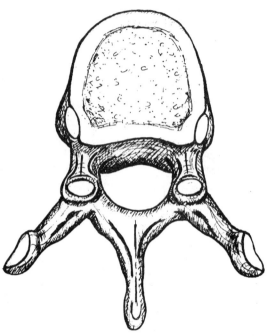

Figure 12.11 *Thoracic vertebra. (From Norkin, CC, and Levangie, PK: Joint Structure and Function: A Comprehensive Analysis, ed 2, FA Davis, Philadelphia, 1992, p 131, with permission.)*

COSTOVERTEBRAL JOINT   Transverse process   Body
Vertebral foramen

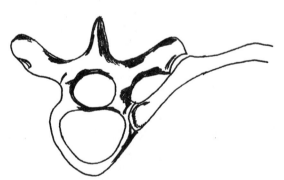

Figure 12.12   *Costovertebral joints.*

TRUE RIBS

FALSE RIBS

FLOATING RIBS

STERNUM

COSTAL CARTILAGE

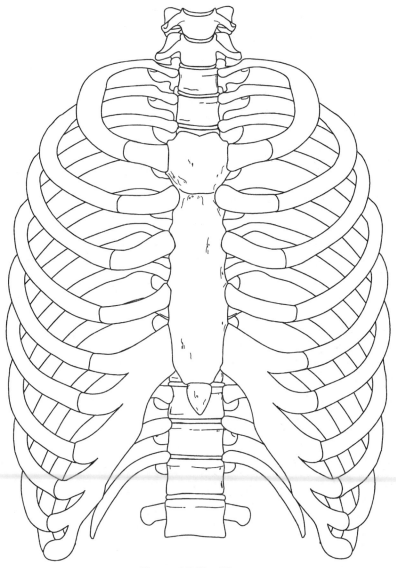

Figure 12.13 *Rib cage.*

PELVIS   Iliac crest   Pubic symphysis

ASIS

PSIS

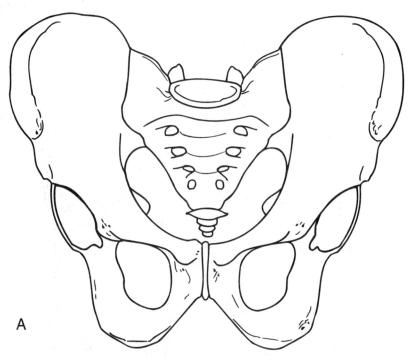

A

Figure 12.14   (A) Anterior view.

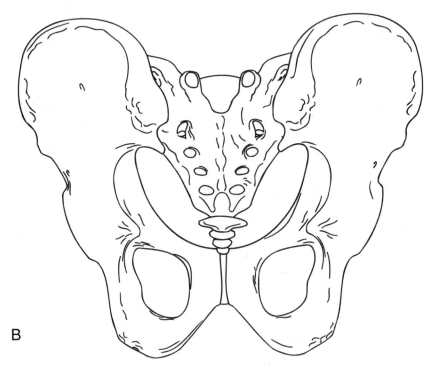

B

Figure 12.14   (B) Posterior view.

3. On the drawing, indicate the locations of the major vertebral structures.

Body   Transverse process   Supraspinal ligament
Spinous process   Interspinous ligament
Anterior longitudinal ligament   Ligamentum flavum
Posterior longitudinal ligament   Intervertebral disk

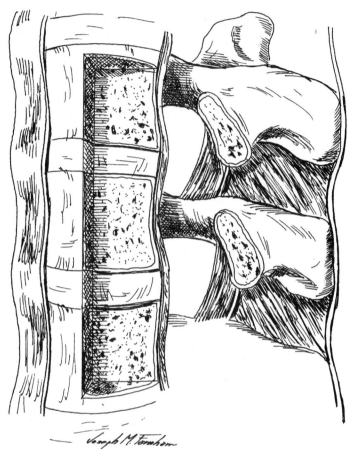

Figure 12.15   *Vertebral ligaments. (From Norkin, CC, and Levangie, PK: Joint Structure and Function: A Comprehensive Analysis, ed 2, FA Davis, Philadelphia, 1992, p 135, with permission.)*

4. On the drawings,

A. Label the origin and insertion of the muscles listed.
Color the origin in red and the insertion in blue.

B. Join the origin and insertion to show the muscle belly.

STERNOCLEIDOMASTOID

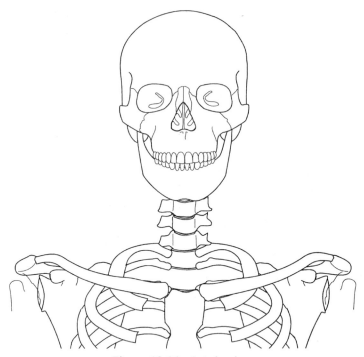

Figure 12.16   *Anterior view.*

SCALENES   Anterior   Posterior   Middle

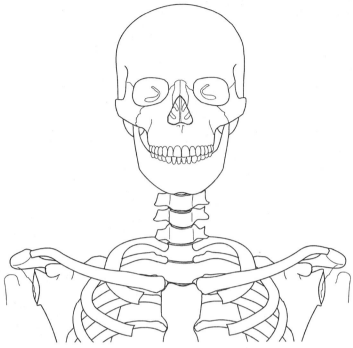

Figure 12.17   *Anterior view.*

SPLENIUS CAPITIS

SPLENIUS CERVICIS

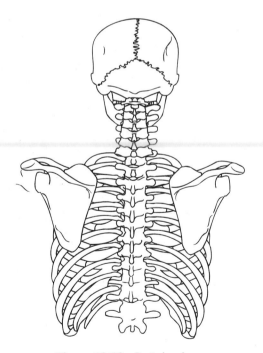

Figure 12.18   *Posterior view.*

RECTUS ABDOMINIS

TRANSVERSE ABDOMINIS

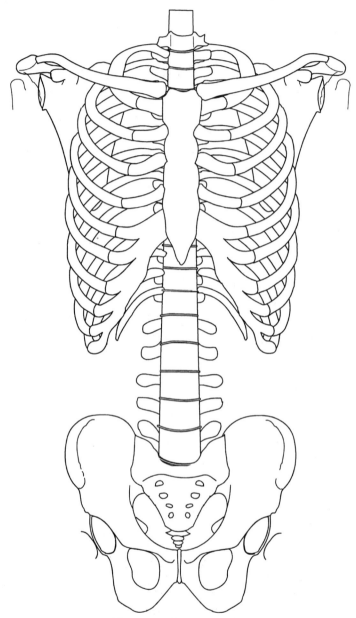

Figure 12.19 *Anterior view.*

EXTERNAL OBLIQUE

INTERNAL OBLIQUE

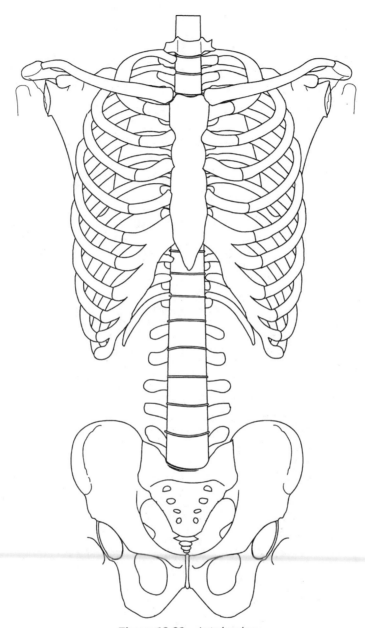

Figure 12.20 *Anterior view.*

ERECTOR SPINAE

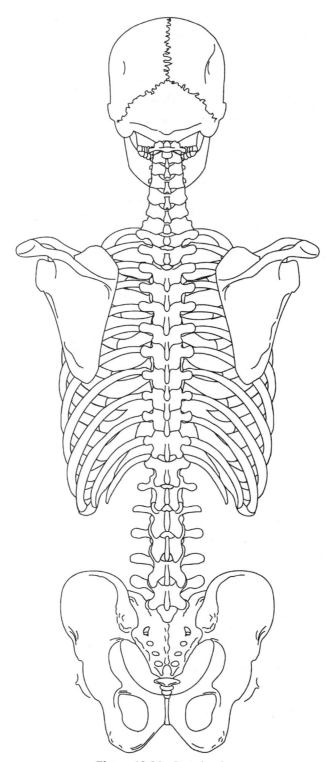

Figure 12.21 *Posterior view.*

TRANSVERSOSPINALIS

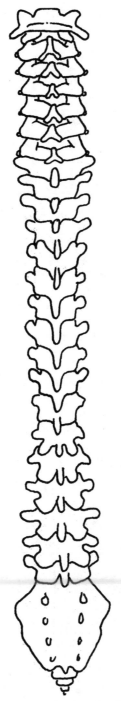

Figure 12.22 *Posterior view.*

INTERSPINALES

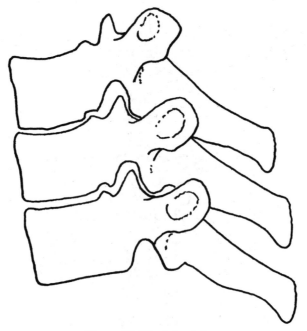

Figure 12.23   *Lateral view.*

INTERTRANSVERSARI

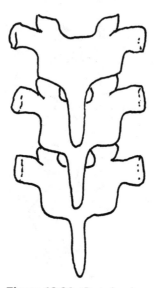

Figure 12.24   *Posterior view.*

QUADRATUS LUMBORUM

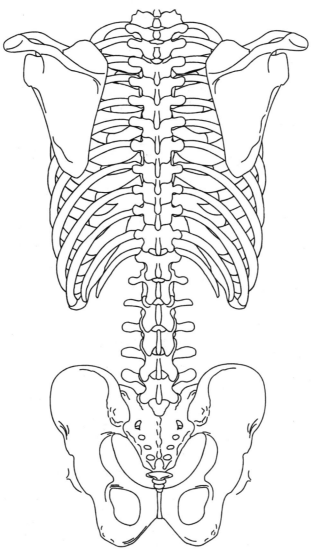

Figure 12.25 *Posterior view.*

DIAPHRAGM

EXTERNAL INTERCOSTALS

INTERNAL INTERCOSTALS

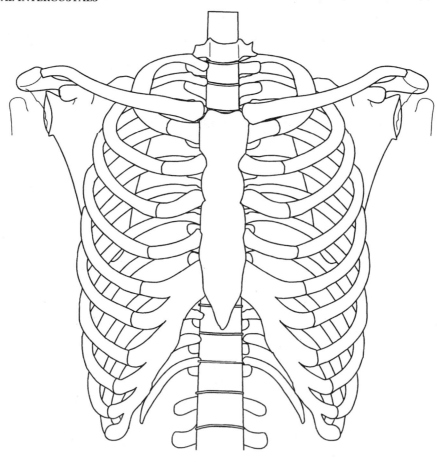

Figure 12.26 *Anterior view.*

5. Define the following terms:

Facet: _____

Facet joint: _____

_____

_____

Demifacet: _____

_____

6. For each joint listed, indicate the motion(s) available.

Joint	Flexion	Extension	Rotation	Lateral Bending
ATLANTO-OCCIPITAL				
ATLANTO-AXIAL				
INTERVERTEBRAL				

7. For each region of the spine, indicate the movement(s) that have the greatest range of motion.

Spinal Region	Flexion/Extension	Lateral Bending	Rotation
CERVICAL			
THORACIC			
LUMBAR			

8. What determines the motion available at each spinal region?_____

_____

9. For each motion listed, check the muscle(s) that performs that motion.

Motion	Sternocleidomastoid	Scalene	Splenius capitis	Splenius cervicis	Erector spinae	Transversospinalis	Interspinales	Intertransversari	Quadratus lumborum
FLEXION									
HYPEREXTENSION									
LATERAL BENDING									
ROTATION									

Motion	Rectus abdominis	External oblique	Internal oblique	Transverse abdominis	Diaphragm	Internal intercostals	External intercostals
FLEXION							
HYPEREXTENSION							
LATERAL BENDING							
ROTATION							
COMPRESS ABDOMEN							
ELEVATE RIBS							
DEPRESS RIBS							
INSPIRATION							
EXPIRATION							

10. What is the name of the vertebral opening that contains the spinal cord? _____

_____

11. What is the name of the vertebral opening through which the nerve root passes? _____

_____

12. The opening identified in question 11 is formed by which structures? _____

_____

13. What is the name of the vertebral opening through which the vertebral artery passes?_____

_____

14. Which portion of the vertebra supports the majority of the body weight? _____

_____

15. Which portion of the vertebra determines the type and amount of motions allowed?_____

_____

16. Ribs attach to vertebra in which region of the vertebral column?_____
    With what process of the vertebra does the rib articulate? _____
    What bony landmarks on the body of the vertebra are points of articulation for the ribs?

    _____

17. As you inhale, in which direction does the rib cage move? _____
    As you exhale, in which direction does the rib cage move? _____

18. For each muscle listed, indicate the phase of respiration and type of respiration to which it contributes.

Muscles	*Inspiration*			*Expiration*	
	Quiet	Deep	Forced	Deep	Forced
INTERNAL INTERCOSTALS					
EXTERNAL INTERCOSTALS					
DIAPHRAGM					
INTERNAL OBLIQUE					
EXTERNAL OBLIQUE					
STERNOCLEIDOMASTOID					
SCALENI					
LEVATOR SCAPULA					
LEVATOR COSTORUM					
SERRATUS POSTERIOR SUPERIOR					
SERRATUS POSTERIOR INFERIOR					
UPPER TRAPEZIUS					
RHOMBOIDS					
PECTORALIS MINOR					
RECTUS ABDOMINIS					
QUADRATUS LUMBORUM					
TRANSVERSE ABDOMINIS					

LAB ACTIVITIES
NECK, TRUNK, AND RESPIRATION

1. Observe from the posterior view, the range of motion, and the shape of the curve of each spinal region as your partner performs spinal flexion, extension, rotation, and lateral bending to each side.

2. On the skeleton, anatomical models, and at least one partner, locate, palpate, and observe the structures described below. The reference position is the anatomical position. Having pictures for reference is helpful when trying to find the structures. Not all structures can be palpated.

   Cervical spine: The cervical spine consists of the first seven vertebrae. Palpate the spinous processes along the midline of the neck.

       Atlas: The first cervical vertebra. It articulates with the skull and the axis. This is palpated just below the skull.

       Axis: The second cervical vertebra.

       Dens: Also called the odontoid process. It is the large vertical projection located anteriorly on the axis. This cannot be palpated.

       C7: Also called the vertebra prominens because it is the largest spinous process. It is easily palpated at the base of the neck when the neck is flexed.

       Ligamentum nuchae: Located superficially between the skull and C7. Palpated in the midline of the cervical spine. Having your partner flex the neck makes the ligament taut and easier to palpate.

       Transverse foramen: Openings in the transverse processes of the cervical vertebra. These cannot be palpated.

   Thoracic spine: The thoracic spine consists of the next 12 vertebrae. Palpate the spinous processes along the midline.

       Costal facets: Located superiorly and inferiorly on the sides of the bodies and on the transverse processes of the thoracic vertebrae. These are the sites of the articulations of the ribs with the vertebrae. These cannot be palpated.

   Lumbar spine: The lumbar spine consists of the next five vertebrae. Palpate the spinous processes along the midline.

   Sacral spine: The sacral spine consists of the last five vertebrae. These vertebrae are fused together. Palpate the base of the spine between the iliums.

   Kyphosis: From the lateral view, the concave shape of the thoracic and sacral spine.

   Lordosis: From the lateral view, the convex shape of the cervical and lumbar spine.

   Skull: The skeleton of the head. Also called the cranium.

       Occipital bone: Posterior inferior part of the skull. The general area of the occipital bone can be palpated.

       Foramen magnum: Opening in the skull through which the spinal cord enters the cranium. This cannot be palpated.

       Condyles: Located inferiorly on the occipital bone on either side of the foramen magnum. These cannot be palpated.

       Temporal bone: Located on the lateral aspect of the skull. This can be palpated on the lateral aspect of the skull just above the ear.

Mastoid process: Bony prominence located behind the ear. Palpate just posterior to the ear.

Vertebrae: Except for the first two vertebrae, the vertebrae generally have the same characteristics:

Body: The anterior rounded weight-bearing portion of the vertebrae. The first two vertebrae do not have a body. The bodies become progressively larger from the cervical region to the sacral region. The body cannot be palpated.

Neural arch: The posterior portion of the vertebrae consisting of the transverse and spinous processes and the lamina. Also called the vertebral arch. These cannot be palpated.

Pedicle: The bony bridge between the body and the neural arch. These cannot be palpated.

Lamina: The bony bridge between the transverse and spinous processes. These cannot be palpated.

Transverse process: The lateral projections at the union of the lamina and pedicle. Palpate on the lateral aspect of the vertebra.

Vertebral notches: Depressions on the superior and inferior surfaces of the pedicle. These cannot be palpated.

Intervertebral foramen: Opening formed by the superior vertebral notch of one vertebrae and the inferior vertebral notch of the vertebra above it. These cannot be palpated.

Articular process: Projections on both the superior and inferior surfaces of the lamina. Superior articular processes face posteriorly or medially. Inferior articular processes face anteriorly or laterally. These cannot be palpated.

Spinous process: The posterior midline projection of the neural arch. These are palpated over the midline of the spine.

Intervertebral disk: Located between the bodies of adjacent vertebrae. These cannot be palpated.

Annulus fibrosus: The outer portion of the intervertebral disk. This cannot be palpated.

Nucleus pulposus: The pulpy gelatinous center portion of the intervertebral disk. This cannot be palpated.

3. Locate the muscles listed below on the skeleton and on at least one partner.

A. Locate the origin and insertion of the muscle on the skeleton.

B. Stretch a large rubber band taut by placing one end at the origin and the other end at the insertion of the muscle on the skeleton.

C. Perform the motion that muscle does and observe how the rubber band becomes less taut and shorter, similar to the muscle shortening as it contracts.

D. Perform the opposite motion and observe how the rubber band becomes more taut and longer, similar to the muscle lengthening as it is stretched.

E. After locating the muscle on the skeleton, locate the muscle on your partner. The position described for locating the muscle on your partner is the manual muscle test position for a fair or better grade of muscle strength. Not all origins, insertions, and muscle bellies can be palpated.

F. When possible, palpate the origin, insertion, and muscle belly of each muscle by:

1) Placing your fingers on the origin and insertion and asking your partner to contract the muscle.

2) Moving your fingers from the origin to the insertion over the contracting muscle.

3) Asking your partner to relax the muscle and again moving your fingers from the origin to the insertion over the muscle.

SUPINE POSITION

Sternocleidomastoid: Located superficially on the anterior and lateral neck.

Origin:	Sternum and medial end of the clavicle.
Insertion:	Mastoid process.
Action:	Bilateral: Flex the head and neck.
	Unilateral: Laterally bend the neck to the same side and rotate the head to the opposite side.
	Accessory muscle of respiration.
Palpate:	Palpate the anterolateral neck from just under the ear to either side of the sternoclavicular joint.

Scaleni: Located on the lateral aspect of the neck and partially deep to the sternocleidomastoid muscle.

Origin:	Anterior: Transverse processes of C3–6.
	Middle: Transverse processes of C2–7.
	Posterior: Transverse processes of C4–6.
Insertion:	Anterior and middle: First rib.
	Posterior: Second rib.
Action:	Bilateral: Flex the head and neck.
	Unilateral: Laterally bend the head and neck.
	Accessory muscles of respiration.
Palpate:	On the lateral aspect of the neck between the sternocleidomastoid anteriorly at the upper trapezius posteriorly. Palpate while partner takes a deep breath. Differentiating among the three parts is difficult.

Rectus abdominis: Located superficially near the midline of the abdomen.

Origin:	Pubis.
Insertion:	Costal cartilages of the fifth to seventh ribs.
Action:	Flex the trunk by lifting the head and shoulders off the table.
	Accessory muscles of respiration.
Palpate:	Along the midline of the abdomen from the pubis to the distal sternum while partner lifts the head and shoulders off of the table.

External oblique: Located superficially on the anterior lateral abdomen.

Origin:	Ribs 4–12.
Insertion:	Iliac crest.
Action:	Flex and rotate the trunk to the opposite side by lifting the head and shoulders off the table.
	Accessory muscles of respiration.
Palpate:	On the left anterior lateral abdomen. To palpate the left external oblique, raise the left shoulder up and toward the right.

Internal oblique: Located deep to the external oblique muscle.

Origin:	Inguinal ligament, iliac crest, and thoracolumbar fascia.
Insertion:	Lower ribs, nine to twelve, and the abdominal aponeurosis.
Action:	Flex and rotate the trunk to the same side by lifting the head and shoulders off the table.
	Accessory muscles of respiration.
Palpate:	On the left anterior lateral abdomen. To palpate the left internal oblique, raise the right shoulder up and toward the left.

Transverse abdominis: Located deep to the oblique muscles.

Origin:	Inguinal ligament, iliac crest, thoracolumbar fascia, and the last six ribs.
Insertion:	Abdominal aponeurosis and linea alba.
Action:	Compress the abdomen. Accessory muscle of respiration.
Palpate:	Palpation is not possible.

Quadratus lumborum: Located deep to the erector spinae.

Origin:	Iliac crest.
Insertion:	Twelfth rib and the transverse processes of L2–5.
Action:	Trunk lateral bending. "Hike" the pelvis. Accessory muscle of respiration.
Palpate:	Palpation is not possible.

Diaphragm: Located deep to the lower ribs.

Origin:	Xiphoid process, ribs, and lumbar vertebrae.
Insertion:	Central tendon.
Action:	Inspiration.
Palpate:	Palpation is not possible.

External intercostal: Located superficially between the ribs anteriorly.

Origin:	Rib above.
Insertion:	Rib below.
Action:	Inspiration, elevate ribs.
Palpate:	Between ribs anteriorly.

Internal intercostal: Located deep to the external intercostal muscle.

Origin:	Rib below.
Insertion:	Rib above.
Action:	Expiration, depress ribs.
Palpate:	Palpation is not possible.

PRONE POSITION

Splenius capitis: Located superficially on the posterior neck.

Origin:	Lower half of the nuchal ligament and spinous processes of C7–T3.
Insertion:	Lateral occipital bone and mastoid process.
Action:	Bilateral: Extend head. Unilateral: Rotate head to same side.
Palpate:	On the posterior upper lateral aspect of the neck.

Splenius cervicis: Located superficially on the posterior neck.

Origin:	Spinous processes of T3–T6.
Insertion:	Transverse processes of C1–C3.
Action:	Bilateral: Extend head and neck. Unilateral: Rotate head to same side.
Palpate:	On the posterior upper lateral aspect of the neck.

Erector spinae: Includes three groups of muscles: spinalis, longissimus, and iliocostalis. Located posteriorly and deep to the shoulder girdle muscles.

Origin: Spinous processes, transverse processes, and posterior ribs from the occiput to the sacrum and ilium.

Insertion: Spinous processes, transverse processes, and posterior ribs from the occiput to the sacrum and ilium.

Action: Bilateral: Extend the trunk.
Unilateral: Lateral bending of the trunk.

Palpate: In the thoracic and lumbar area on either side of the spine, while raising the shoulders off the table.

Transversospinalis: Includes three muscle groups: rotatores, multifidus, and semispinalis. Located posteriorly and deep to the erector spinae.

Origin: Transverse processes.

Insertion: Spinous processes of the vertebra above.

Action: Bilateral: Extend the trunk.
Unilateral: Rotate the trunk to the opposite side.

Palpate: Palpation is not possible.

Interspinales: Located deep.

Origin: Spinous process of vertebra below.

Insertion: Spinous process of vertebra above.

Action: Extend trunk.

Palpate: Palpation is not possible.

Intertransversarii: Located deep.

Origin: Transverse process of vertebra below.

Insertion: Transverse process of vertebra above.

Action: Bend trunk laterally.

Palpate: Palpation is not possible.

4. Have a partner lie supine on a table with the hands on the shoulders and the legs extended. Place one hand on the small of your partner's back and the other hand on the abdominal muscles.

A. When your partner presses his or her low back into the table, which muscles are the agonists?_____

B. Which muscles are the antagonists?_____

C. What is this motion called? _____

D. If your partner is unable to press his or her low back to the table, which muscles may be too short (tight)? _____

E. If your partner is unable to press his or her low back to the table, which muscles may be too long (weak)? _____

5. In the standing position, slide your left hand down the side of your leg, thereby bringing your shoulder closer to your knee.

    A. What motion did you perform?_____

    B. Which muscle(s) performed the motion? _____

    _____

6. In the standing position, lift your foot off the floor while keeping your hip and knee extended.

    A. What motion did you perform?_____

    B. Which muscle(s) performed the motion? _____

7. Starting in the supine position, raise your head off the table.

    A. What motion did you perform?_____

    B. Which muscle(s) act as stabilizers to permit lifting the head? _____

    C. What is being stabilized and why? _____

    _____

    _____

8. Starting in the supine position, raise your head and shoulders off the table.

    A. What motion did you perform?_____

    B. Which muscle(s) performed the motion? _____

9. Starting in the supine position, raise your right shoulder off the table and toward your left knee.

    A. What motion did you perform?_____

    B. Which muscle(s) performed the motion? _____

10. Starting in the supine position, perform a *bilateral straight leg raise*, lifting your heels about 10 inches off the table.

    NOTE: Do not perform this activity if you have low back problems.

    A. What motion did you perform?_____

    B. What position does the lumbar spine assume during this activity? _____

    C. What muscles should act as stabilizers during this activity? _____

11. Sit-ups are often included in general exercise programs.

Perform a sit-up with your legs straight.

Perform a sit-up with your hips and knees flexed so your feet are flat on the floor.

Perform an abdominal curl (partial sit-up).

A. What is the purpose of performing a sit-up or abdominal curl? _____

B. Is there a difference in effectiveness when a sit-up is performed with the legs straight compared to with the hips and knees flexed? _____

C. Is there a benefit to performing a sit-up rather than an abdominal curl? Explain your answer.

_____

_____

12. Observe your partner breathe quietly and while taking deep breaths—tell him or her to avoid hyperventilating. Perform in sitting and supine positions. Describe what you observed._____

_____

_____

13. Diagram the lever that describes the activity at the lumbosacral joint when in standing your partner performs a trunk curl. Do not bend at the hips and knees.

A. On the figure, label the Xs that represent the axis, muscle, and gravity, and identify the specific joint and muscle group.

B. Make arrows out of the vertical lines to indicate the direction of the movement, the direction of the pull of the muscle, and the direction of gravity.

C. Identify the muscle and gravity as either *force* or *resistance*.

X   X   X   Direction of movement

14. Analyze the activity of the lumbosacral joint diagrammed in question 13 by answering the following questions.

   A. Which joint motion is being analyzed?_____

   B. Is the movement moving with gravity or against gravity? _____

   C. Is there any external force giving resistance to the trunk? _____

   D. Which major muscle group is the agonist?_____

   E. Which major muscle group is the antagonist?_____

   F. Is the muscle acting to overcome gravity or to slow down gravity?_____

   G. Is the agonist performing a concentric or an eccentric contraction?_____

   H. Is this an open or closed kinetic chain activity? _____

15. Diagram the lever that describes the activity at the lumbosacral joint when your partner returns to a standing position after performing a trunk curl.

   A. On the figure, label the Xs that represent the axis, muscle, and gravity, and identify the specific joint and muscle group.

   B. Make arrows out of the vertical lines to indicate the direction of the movement, the direction of the pull of the muscle, and the direction of gravity.

   C. Identify the muscle and gravity as either *force* or *resistance*.

X	X	X	Direction of movement

16. Analyze the activity of the lumbosacral joint diagrammed in question 15 by answering the following questions.

   A. Which joint motion is being analyzed?_____

   B. Is the movement moving with gravity or against gravity? _____

   C. Is there any external force giving resistance to the trunk? _____

   D. Which major muscle group is the agonist?_____

   E. Which major muscle group is the antagonist?_____

   F. Is the muscle acting to overcome gravity or slow down gravity? _____

   G. Is the agonist performing a concentric or an eccentric contraction?_____

   H. Is this an open or closed kinetic chain activity? _____

POST-LAB QUESTIONS
NECK, TRUNK, AND RESPIRATION

After you have completed the Worksheets and the Lab Activities, answer the following questions without using your books or notes. When finished, check your answers.

1. Identify the other terms for which each of the following bones or landmarks are known:

   A. The dens: _____

   B. The seventh cervical vertebra: _____

   C. The first cervical vertebra: _____

   D. The second cervical vertebra: _____

   E. The neural arch: _____

2. Which vertebra does not have a spinous process or a body? _____

3. C1 articulates with which landmark of which skull bone? _____

4. Name one characteristic that distinguishes one group of vertebrae from the others.

   Cervical: _____

   Thoracic: _____

   Lumbar: _____

5. How many pairs of ribs are there? _____

6. Complete the following table of information about the ribs.

Name	Number	Location	Attachment to the sternum
True			Direct via costal cartilage
	3		
		11th and 12th ribs	

7. Torticollis is a result of shortening or spasm of the sternocleidomastoid muscle. What position does the head assume when the left sternocleidomastoid muscle is involved? _____

_____

8. If the curvatures of the spine were fixed, which muscles and ligaments would be short and which long at each region listed in the table?

Spinal region	Shortened	Lengthened
CERVICAL		
THORACIC		
LUMBAR		

9. On each of the following drawings, place arrows to represent the muscles that maintain the position of the pelvis. Label the arrows with the muscle each represents.

A. Pelvis level

B. Anterior pelvic tilt

C. Posterior pelvic tilt

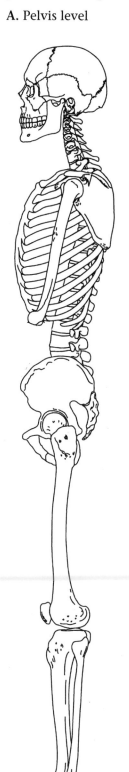

Figure 12.27 *Lateral view.*

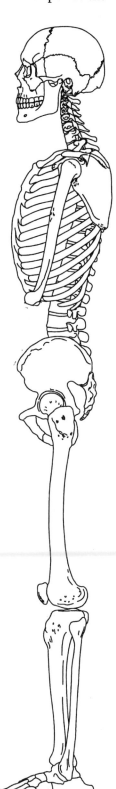

Figure 12.28 *Lateral view.*

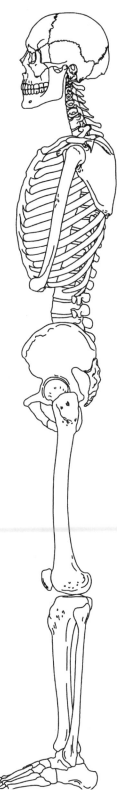

Figure 12.29 *Lateral view.*

10. For a person with a fixed anterior or posterior pelvic tilt, identify which muscles are in shortened positions and which are in lengthened positions.

Position	Shortened	Lengthened
ANTERIOR PELVIC TILT		
POSTERIOR PELVIC TILT		

13

POSTURE
An Introduction

Posture is observed and compared to an ideal or standard. A plumb line suspended from the ceiling or a posture grid behind the person is used as a point of reference during posture assessment. Described below is the ideal relationship of joints and structures in relation to the plumb line used when performing a posture observation. When an individual has ideal alignment, the *stress* on structures and the amount of muscle energy required to maintain posture are reduced.

ANTERIOR VIEW

The plumb line is essentially aligned over the midsagittal plane of the body and therefore divides the body into two equal halves (Fig. 13.1). In addition to dividing the body into two equal halves, the following are also considered part of ideal alignment.

Feet: slightly toeing out
Ankles: normal arch in feet
Knees: level and not bowed or knock-kneed
Hips: level, both ASISs in same plane
Sternum: centered
Shoulders: level and not elevated or depressed
Head and face: head not flexed or hyperextended

POSTERIOR VIEW

The plumb line is essentially aligned over the midsagittal plane of the body and therefore divides the body into two equal halves (Fig. 13.2). In addition to dividing the body into two equal halves, the following are also considered part of ideal alignment.

Ankles: calcaneus straight
Knees: level and not bowed or knock-kneed
Hips: level, both PSISs in same plane
Spinous processes: centered
Shoulders: level and not elevated or depressed
Head: head not flexed or hyperextended

LATERAL VIEW

The plumb line is aligned over the frontal plane that is slightly in front of the lateral malleolus (Fig. 13.3). The plumb line passes:

Ankle: slightly anterior to lateral malleolus
Knee: slightly anterior to axis of knee joint (slightly posterior to patella)
Hip: slightly posterior to axis of hip joint (through the greater trochanter)
Lumbar spine: through the bodies of the lumbar spine
Thoracic spine: anterior to vertebral bodies
Shoulder: tip of the acromion process
External auditory meatus: through the ear lobe
Head: slightly posterior to the apex

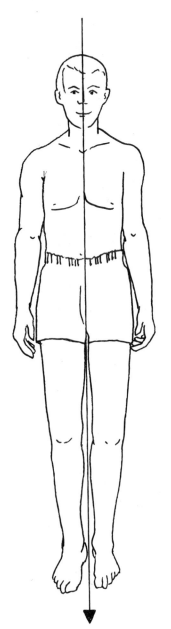

Figure 13.1 *Posture, anterior view.*

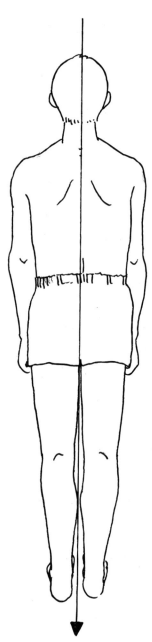

Figure 13.2 *Posture, posterior view.*

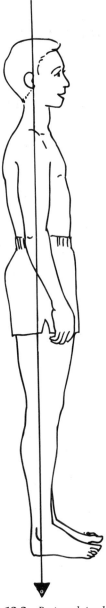

Figure 13.3 *Posture, lateral view.*

WORKSHEETS
POSTURE

Complete the following questions prior to lab class.

1. Which hip and trunk muscles are responsible for maintaining the pelvis level in the frontal plane?

   _____

   _____

2. A. Another name for "knock-knees" is _____ in which the distal segment (foot) is aligned toward/away (circle one) from the midline.

   B. Another name for "bowlegs" is _____ in which the distal segment (foot) is aligned toward/away (circle one) from the midline.

3. List the four normal curves of the spine and identify whether they are concave or convex as viewed posteriorly.

   Curve   *Concave/Convex*

   _____   _____

   _____   _____

   _____   _____

   _____   _____

   _____   _____

LAB ACTIVITIES
POSTURE

1. **A.** Observe from the posterior view five partners who are right-handed and five (or as many as are available) partners who are left-handed.

   B. Determine which shoulder, the dominant or nondominant shoulder, of the majority of the members of each group is higher.

   C. Can you generalize as to whether the dominant shoulder is high or low? _____

   _____

2. In groups of three, observe your partners' posture from the anterior, posterior, and both lateral views using a plumb line. Each individual in the group is to be the subject, the lead observer, and the assistant observer. Record the deviations from the normal observed in each view. Do not get too detailed. Because some individuals become faint from standing still for a long time due to pooling of blood, work in a timely manner and provide the subject with opportunities to walk around between views.

   Suspend a string with a weight (plumb line) from the ceiling. In all views, position the subject's feet 2 to 4 inches apart with the heels even and the toes pointing slightly outward close to the plumb line but so they will not touch the plumb line when they sway. For the anterior and posterior views, the plumb line should divide the space between the feet equally. In the lateral views, the plumb line is positioned slightly anterior to the lateral malleolus. When the feet are aligned correctly, the subject's body should line up correctly with the plumb line unless the individual has a postural deviation.

   The following form can be used to record your observations.

Anterior view

   Ankles: _____

   Knees: _____

   Hips: _____

   Sternum: _____

   Shoulders: _____

   Face: _____

Posterior view

   Ankles: _____

   Knees: _____

   Hips: _____

   Spinous processes: _____

   Shoulders: _____

   Head: _____

Right lateral view

Ankle:_____

Knee: _____

Hip: _____

Lumbar spine: _____

Thoracic spine:_____

Acromion process: _____

Ear lobe: _____

Top of head:_____

Left lateral view

Ankle:_____

Knee: _____

Hip: _____

Lumbar spine: _____

Thoracic spine:_____

Acromion process: _____

Ear lobe: _____

Top of head:_____

POST-LAB QUESTIONS
POSTURE

After you have completed the Lab Activities, answer the following questions without using your books or notes. When finished, check your answers.

1. When performing a posture observation, which view is best to determine that the individual being observed:

    A. Lacks full knee extension? _____

    B. Has lateral bending of the trunk?_____

    C. Has forward shoulders?_____

2. What postural deviations would result from the right lower extremity being longer than the left?

    _____

    _____

    _____

3. When a posture observation was performed, the following deviations were noted in the lateral view: Anterior pelvic tilt, increased lumbar lordosis, and a protruding abdomen.

    A. Which muscles should be evaluated to determine whether they are too short? _____

    _____

    B. Which muscles should be evaluated to determine whether they are too long?_____

    _____

14

GAIT
An Introduction

The positions of the hip, knee, ankle, and toes have been described for each phase of gait for the Rancho Los Amigos (RLA) approach to gait assessment. These positions are as follows:

INITIAL CONTACT

Hip: 25° flexion
Knee: 0°
Ankle: 0°
Toes: 0°

LOADING RESPONSE

Hip: 25° flexion
Knee: 15° flexion
Ankle: 10° plantar flexion
Toes: 0°

MIDSTANCE

Hip: 0°
Knee: 0°
Ankle: 5° dorsiflexion
Toes: 0°

TERMINAL STANCE

Hip: 20° hyperextension
Knee: 0°
Ankle: 10° dorsiflexion
Toes: 30° metatarsal phalangeal (MTP) extension

PRESWING

Hip: 0°
Knee: 40° flexion
Ankle: 20° plantar flexion
Toes: 60° MTP extension

INITIAL SWING

Hip: 15° flexion
Knee: 60° flexion
Ankle: 10° plantar flexion
Toes: 0°

MIDSWING

Hip: 25° flexion
Knee: 25° flexion
Ankle: 0°
Toes: 0°

TERMINAL SWING

Hip: 25° flexion
Knee: 0°
Ankle: 0°
Toes: 0°

Reference: Observational Gait Analysis Handbook by The Pathokinesiology Service and The Physical Therapy Department of Rancho Los Amigos Medical Center, Downey, Calif, 1993.

Student's Name _____ Date Due _____

WORKSHEETS
GAIT

Complete the following questions prior to lab class.

1. Match the following terms and definitions. There may be more than one answer.

   _____ Distance between heel strike of one foot
   and heel strike of the other foot

   _____ Side-to-side distance between footprints

   _____ Distance between heel strike of one foot
   and heel strike of the same foot

   _____ That part of the gait cycle when the foot
   is in contact with the ground

   _____ That part of the gait cycle when the foot
   is not in contact with the ground

   A. Stance phase
   B. Stride length
   C. Step width
   D. Swing phase
   E. Step length
   F. Gait cycle

2. List the components of the stance phase of gait using both the traditional and the RLA
   terminology.

   TRADITIONAL   **RLA**

   _____   _____

   _____   _____

   _____   _____

   _____   _____

   _____   _____

3. List the components of the swing phase of gait using both the traditional and the RLA terminology.

   TRADITIONAL   **RLA**

   _____   _____

   _____   _____

   _____   _____

   _____   _____

   _____   _____

4. Match the phase of gait using the RLA terminology with the position of the joints.

IC—Initial contact　　　　LR—Loading response　　　MSt—Midstance
TSt—Terminal stance　　　PSw—Preswing　　　　　　ISw—Initial swing
MSw—Midswing　　　　　　TSw—Terminal swing

A. Phase: _____

　　Hip:　0°

　　Knee:　0°

　　Ankle: 5° dorsiflexion

　　Toes:　0°

B. Phase: _____

　　Hip:　25° flexion

　　Knee:　0°

　　Ankle: 0°

　　Toes:　0°

C. Phase: _____

　　Hip:　15° flexion

　　Knee: 60° flexion

　　Ankle: 10° plantar flexion

　　Toes:　0°

D. Phase: _____

　　Hip:　25° flexion

　　Knee: 15° flexion

　　Ankle: 10° plantar flexion

　　Toes:　0°

E. Phase: _____

　　Hip:　20° hyperextension

　　Knee:　0°

　　Ankle: 10° dorsiflexion

　　Toes:　30° MTP extension

F. Phase: _____

　　Hip:　25° flexion

　　Knee: 25° flexion

　　Ankle: 0°

　　Toes:　0°

G. Phase: _____

    Hip: 0°

    Knee: 40° flexion

    Ankle: 20° plantar flexion

    Toes: 60° MTP extension

5. For the phase of gait given, indicate which muscles are working at each joint listed.

   A. Phase IC

      Hip: _____

      Knee: _____

      Ankle: _____

   B. Phase LR

      Hip: _____

      Knee: _____

      Ankle: _____

   C. Phase MSt

      Hip: _____

      Knee: _____

      Ankle: _____

   D. Phase TSt

      Hip: _____

      Knee: _____

      Ankle: _____

   E. Phase PSw

      Hip: _____

      Knee: _____

      Ankle: _____

   F. Phase ISw

      Hip: _____

      Knee: _____

      Ankle: _____

   G. Phase MSw

      Hip: _____

      Knee: _____

      Ankle: _____

H. Phase TSw

Hip: _____

Knee: _____

Ankle: _____

6. Identify and label the phase of gait represented by the reference limb, the right lower extremity.

A. _____ *Fig. 14-1*

B. _____ *Fig. 14-2*

C. _____ *Fig. 14-3*

D. _____ *Fig. 14-4*

E. _____ *Fig. 14-5*

F. _____ *Fig. 14-6*

G. _____ *Fig. 14-7*

H. _____ *Fig. 14-8*

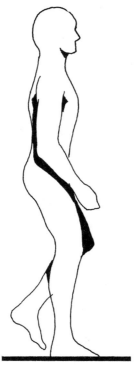

Figure 14.1 *(From Norkin, CC, and Levangie, PK: Joint Structure and Function: A Comprehensive Analysis, ed 2. FA Davis, Philadelphia, 1992, p 453, with permission.)*

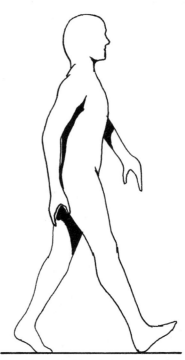

Figure 14.2 *(From Norkin, CC, and Levangie, PK: Joint Structure and Function: A Comprehensive Analysis, ed 2. FA Davis, Philadelphia, 1992, p 453, with permission.)*

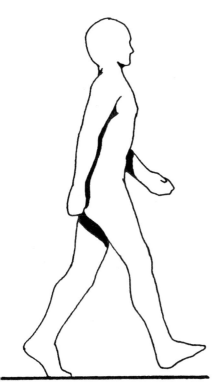

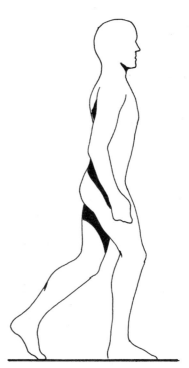

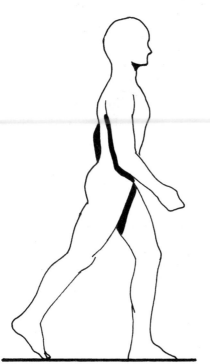

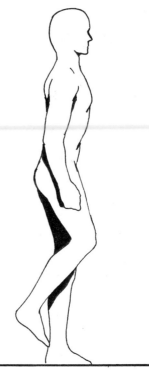

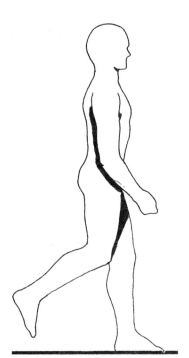

Figure 14.7 *(From Norkin, CC, and Levangie, PK: Joint Structure and Function: A Comprehensive Analysis, ed 2. FA Davis, Philadelphia, 1992, p 455, with permission.)*

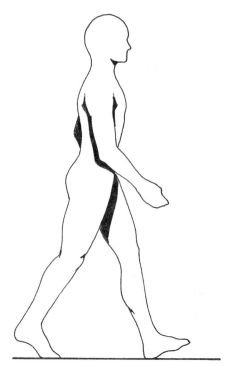

Figure 14.8 *(From Norkin, CC, and Levangie, PK: Joint Structure and Function: A Comprehensive Analysis, ed 2. FA Davis, Philadelphia, 1992, p 454, with permission.)*

LAB ACTIVITIES
GAIT

1. In groups of three, observe the gait of your partners. Each member of the group is to be the subject, the lead evaluator, and the assistant evaluator. The subject is to walk at normal cadence without wearing shoes. Arrange an area large enough so the subject is able to walk at normal speed and the observers have sufficient space to observe and move as needed to observe from the front, back, and each side. As time permits, observe additional individuals walk.

   Initial observation should be of the "whole person" as the individual walks. Note speed and any peculiarities.

   Second observation is to identify when each phase of the gait cycle is occurring: IC, LR, MSt, TSt, PSw, ISw, MSw, and TSw.

   Next, starting with the toes, observe each body segment through all phases of gait and from all views. Compare your observations of your partner to the normal motion that should be occurring in each phase. Indicate in the space if the motion is normal (N), less than normal (↓), or greater than normal (↑).

   A. Phase IC

   Hip: 25° flexion _____

   Knee: 0°   _____

   Ankle: 0°   _____

   Toes: 0°   _____

   B. Phase LR

   Hip: 25° flexion   _____

   Knee: 15° flexion   _____

   Ankle: 10° plantar flexion _____

   Toes: 0°   _____

   C. Phase MSt

   Hip: 0°   _____

   Knee: 0°   _____

   Ankle: 5° dorsiflexion _____

   Toes: 0°   _____

   D. Phase TSt

   Hip: 20° hyperextension _____

   Knee: 0°   _____

   Ankle: 10° dorsiflexion   _____

   Toes: 30° MCP extension _____

E. Phase PSw

Hip: 0°   _____

Knee: 40° flexion   _____

Ankle: 20° plantar flexion   _____

Toes: 60° MTP extension   _____

F. Phase ISw

Hip: 15° flexion   _____

Knee: 60° flexion   _____

Ankle: 10° plantar flexion   _____

Toes: 0°   _____

G. Phase MSw

Hip: 25° flexion _____

Knee: 25° flexion _____

Ankle: 0°   _____

Toes: 0°   _____

H. Phase TSw

Hip: 25° flexion _____

Knee: 0°   _____

Ankle: 0°   _____

Toes: 0°   _____

2. In a group, observe what happens to the components of gait as the individual walking varies cadence from very slow to very fast (do not run). Describe the changes observed.

_____

_____

_____

_____

3. In a group, observe what happens to the components of gait when the individual walking uses a cane, a walker, or a sling on one arm. Describe how the gait changed with each situation.

A. A cane: _____

B. A walker: _____

C. A sling on one arm: _____

POST-LAB QUESTIONS
GAIT

1. Identify the following descriptions of gait phases by giving the traditional terminology and the RLA terminology.

Description	Traditional Terminology	Rancho Los Amigos Terminology
Body weight shock is absorbed.		
Body is farthest ahead of foot.		
Leg begins to advance.		
The foot strikes the ground.		
Period of single limb support.		
Leg is in its shortest position.		
Body height reaches highest point.		
Dorsiflexors contract eccentrically.		
Point just before foot leaves the floor.		
Hamstrings contract eccentrically.		

2. Indicate the direction of movement (flexing or extending) at the joints listed in the phases of gait given below.

   A. Heel strike to foot flat (initial contact to loading response)

      Knee: _____

      Ankle: _____

   B. Foot flat to midstance (loading response to midstance)

      Hip: _____

      Ankle: _____

   C. Heel off (terminal stance)

      Knee: _____

      Ankle: _____

   D. Acceleration to midswing (initial swing to midswing)

      Hip: _____

      Knee: _____

3. In which phases of gait do the following motions occur?

    A. Hip flexion: _____

    B. Knee extension: _____

    C. Ankle dorsiflexion: _____

APPENDIX

DRAWINGS OF THE SKELETON

The following full-body illustrations may be reproduced to provide the student opportunities for additional practice at locating muscles, bones, joints, and other structures.

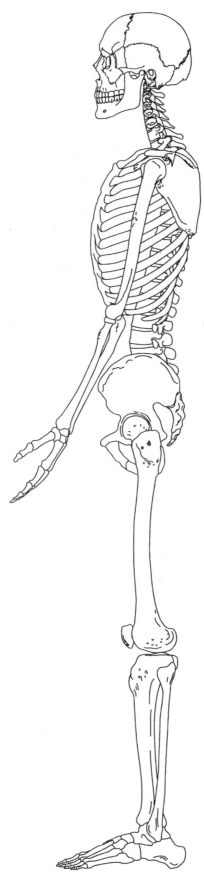

Lateral view.

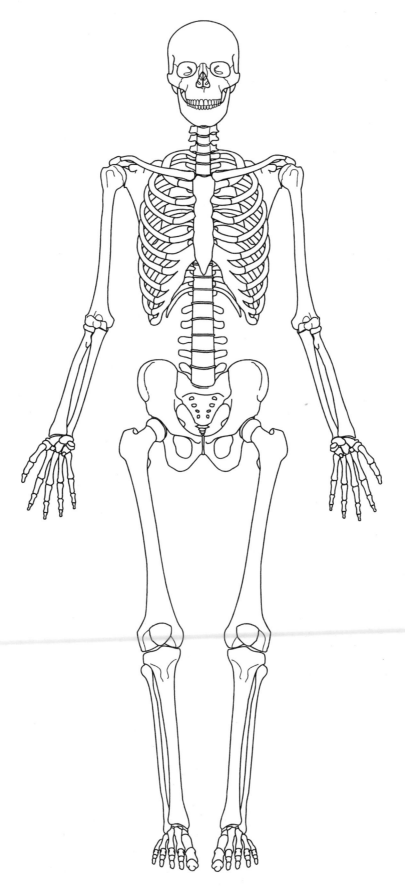

Anterior view.

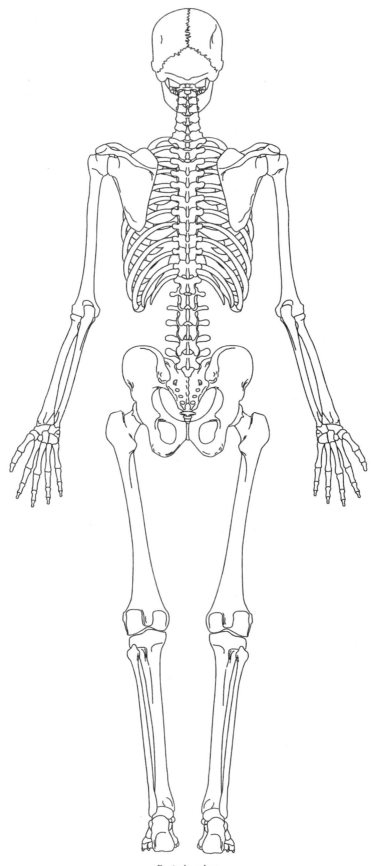

Posterior view.